COMMUNITY CARE: EVALUATION OF THE PROVISION OF MENTAL HEALTH SERVICES

Cyflwynir y llyfr hwn i'r holl gleifian a fu yn Ysbyty Gogledd Cymru.

This book is dedicated to all the former patients of North Wales Hospital.

Community Care: Evaluation of the Provision of Mental Health Services

Edited by
CHARLES CROSBY
MARGARET M. BARRY

Avebury

Aldershot · Brookfield USA · Hong Kong · Singapore · Sydney

Published by
Avebury
Ashgate Publishing Company
Gower House
Croft Road
Aldershot
Hants GU11 3HR
England

Ashgate Publishing Company
Old Post Road
Brookfield
Vermont 05036
USA

British Library Cataloguing in Publication Data

Community Care: Evaluation of the Provision
    of Mental Health Services
    I. Crosby, Charles   II. Barry, Margaret
    362.22094291

ISBN 1 85628 531 6

Library of Congress Catalog Card Number: 94-79825

Printed and bound by Athenæum Press Ltd.,
Gateshead, Tyne & Wear.

Contents

Figures and tables

List of contributors

Margaret M. Barry, M.A., Ph.D. - Lecturer in Psychology, Department of Psychology, Trinity College, Dublin (formerly Deputy Director, Health Services Research Unit).

Michael F. Carter, B.A. - Research Officer, Health Services Research Unit, University College of North Wales, Bangor.

Charles Crosby, B.A. M.Sc., Ph.D., - Director, Health Services Research Unit, University College of North Wales, Bangor.

Rachel Forrester-Jones, B.Sc - Research Student and Part-Time Lecturer, Centre for Social Policy Research and Development, University College of North Wales, Bangor.

Neil Garrod, B.Sc., Ph.D., A.C.T.S. - Professor of Financial Analysis, Department of Accounting and Finance, University of Glasgow (formerly Professor of Accounting, School of Accounting, Banking and Economics, University College of North Wales).

Susan A. Geertshuis, B.A., Ph.D. - Research Fellow, Health Services Research Unit, University College of North Wales, Bangor.

Gordon Grant, B.Sc., M.Sc., Ph.D. - Co-Director, Centre for Social Policy Research and Development, University College of North Wales, Bangor.

David Healy, M.D., M.R.C Psych. - Director of the Academic Sub-Department of Psychological Medicine; Senior Lecturer in Psychological Medicine, University of Wales College of Medicine; Consultant Psychiatrist, Gwynedd Community Trust.

David Mitchell, B.Sc., Ph.D. - Lecturer, Department of Psychology and Sociology, James Cook University of North Queensland, Townsville, Australia (formerly Research Officer, Health Services Research Unit, University College of North Wales).

Sandra Vick, B.A. M.Phil - Research Assistant, Health Economics Research Unit, Department of Public Health, University of Aberdeen (formerly Health Services Research Unit/School of Accounting, Banking and Economics, University College of North Wales).

Brian Williams, B.Sc. - Research Officer, Academic Sub-Department of Psychological Medicine, North Wales Hospital, Denbigh.

Foreword

Professor Fergus Lowe
University College of North Wales

What happens to people who are moved from a large mental hospital, where they have spent many years, to new life-styles and accommodation in community settings? How is their mental health affected by such a move? How are they cared for? What is the impact on their quality of life? These are some of the questions addressed in this book, the publication of which represents the culmination of a sustained research collaboration between members of the Department of Psychology, the Centre for Social Policy Research, and the School of Accounting, Banking and Economics at the University of Wales, Bangor.

In January 1987 Clwyd Health Authority issued a consultative document which outlined a strategy for changing the provision of mental health services in Clwyd over the next ten years. This included a plan for the shifting of almost all mental health services away from the North Wales Hospital site in Denbigh to a range of locally-based residential and day services. It was recognised that a key component in the implementation of this resettlement of long-term residents from the hospital to the community was that it should be suitably monitored and evaluated. To this end Clwyd and Gwynedd Health authorities initiated discussions with the relevant Departments at the University and a programme of research was set in train. That research has since generated valuable contributions to the nationwide process of hospital resettlement, in the form of publications, conference presentations, workshops and seminars. It has given illuminating feedback to frontline workers and managers, and has provided valuable information also to a wider audience of academic, professional and government bodies.

As well as reporting on the continuing evaluation of resettlement, contributors to the book also outline the likely future of services in the community and, most importantly, those who presently use the new mental health services provide their comments. This is as it should be, since their increasing involvement in the shaping of services is a decisive feature of new patterns of provision.

The Department of Health and the Welsh Office in collaboration with the Health Services and Social Services Departments in Clwyd and Gwynedd have supported this project. We are grateful to all who have contributed.

I believe that this book will testify to the value of their efforts, and underline also how much the University has to offer to this vital area of public policy.

Professor C. Fergus Lowe
Head of Department
Department of Psychology,
University College of North Wales

Acknowledgements

Many people have made the research reported here, and the production of this book, possible. The editors would particularly like to thank all the residents and care staff at the North Wales Hospital and in the community care schemes who made the work possible and who contributed time and effort so generously. The authors of the original research proposal (Professor Fergus Lowe, Dr Gordon Grant, Mr John Morrell, Mr Wassim Alladin and Mr Nick Ellis in consultation with the Welsh Office, Department of Health, Clwyd and Gwynedd Health Authorities and Clwyd and Gwynedd Social Services Departments) produced a sound research design from which to work and have continued to support the project generously. Production of the book would not have been possible without the skill and commitment of Mrs Sue Peet, in the early stages, and Mrs Alison Froom, Secretary in the Health Services Research Unit who has been responsible for the production of the final copy. Present and former members of the Health Services Reseach Unit have given valuable support throughout the project.

To these, and many others who have assisted us, our sincere thanks.

Acknowledgements

1 Introduction – Background to the evaluation project

Charles Crosby and Margaret M. Barry

The evaluation project, which is reported in this book, was developed in response to mental health policy and service initiatives in Wales and, in particular, in response to the decision to close the North Wales Hospital, Denbigh. The plan to close the North Wales Hospital (NWH) forms part of an overall policy strategy to transform the mental health services in Wales in line with developments throughout Britain. The Welsh Office document, 'Mental Illness Services: A Strategy for Wales' (May, 1989) sets out the aims and key principles for the development of a comprehensive range of community-based mental health services and facilities throughout Wales which are locally based and will provide effective alternatives to in-patient care. Central funding from the Welsh Office is being made available to promote the changes in the pattern of services at a local level. Each District Health Authority or county is required to produce a joint county plan outlining the development of community services within their district.

In response to the All Wales Strategy, Clwyd Health Authority issued a consultative document in January 1987, outlining proposals for the relocation of almost all mental health services away from the present North Wales Hospital site, and the establishment instead of a range of locally based residential and day services for the various client groups concerned. In addition there was a clear commitment to the development of community-oriented mental health services forged through links with local social services, primary care workers as well as voluntary organisations. Clwyd Health Authority's 1987 consultative document together with subsequent documents such as The Clwyd County Plan for Mental Illness Services (1991) set out the local strategy for the planning, management and implementation of the closure of the North Wales Hospital and the reprovision of services within localities in the county.

Up to 1987 the North Wales Hospital was the main site for the provision of care for people with mental heath problems in the counties of Gwynedd and Clwyd. The hospital, located in open countryside on a site of about 45 acres on the edge of Denbigh, was opened in 1848 with 200 beds to serve the North Wales catchment area. Like many other psychiatric institutions established at this time, the hospital developed a pattern of providing mainly long-term custodial care. There followed a rapid increase in the in-patient population coupled with a low discharge rate. In 1865 another 200 beds were added to accommodate this pattern of admission. The same number again were added in 1891. Another 400 beds were provided in 1914 and this brought the total to 1,000 beds to serve a population of 480,000 in the North Wales area. During subsequent years the hospital population grew to a maximum of 1,409 in 1964 which resulted in considerable overcrowding. Given the general public concern in relation to the detention of large numbers of people in psychiatric hospitals at this time, there followed a shift in policy in North Wales towards earlier discharge which resulted in the population of the hospital being reduced progressively to 661 patients by 1970.

This pattern of change was typical of developments in many areas of England and Wales at this time. The nine psychiatric hospitals throughout Wales underwent a significant change in the pattern of admissions and durations of stay, with the number of in-patients falling from over 6,000 in the 1970s to under 4,000 in 1987. The developing pattern was one of a drop in the number of long-stay patients, with short-term admissions and re-admissions for most patients. By 1987, when the Clwyd Health Authority consultative document was issued, there were some 546 beds available at North Wales Hospital together with 56 long-stay beds at Pool Park, Ruthin (an annexe to the NWH), 10 EMI assessment beds at the Maelor Hospital, Wrexham and 40 acute psychiatric beds at Ysbyty Gwynedd, a general hospital in Bangor. Of the beds at Pool Park and the North Wales Hospital some 44.8% were occupied by long-stay residents with 22.6% of the hospital population being 65 years or over. The North Wales Hospital site is now set for closure in 1995, with the bulk of mental health services being transferred to community-based facilities. From its maximum of 1,409 beds in 1964, numbers have now dropped to below 300 for the first time in over 120 years.

In view of the scale of the changes planned and the need to ensure that adequate community services were in place before the process of hospital run down went ahead, it was recognised by both policy makers and service providers that a key component in the successful implementation of this policy in Wales was the monitoring and evaluation of the process of hospital closure. A number of resettlement projects in Britain had been criticised for their failure to improve or maintain the quality of life of patients when discharged to the community. There was also an awareness that the policy of deinstitutionalisation, both in the USA and Britain, generated a considerable amount of controversy and debate and that

2

professional opinion remained divided concerning the feasibility of closing the large mental hospitals and replacing them with locally based community services. Doubts were also being raised throughout Britain about the capacity of the new community services to provide a truly comprehensive service to people with serious mental health problems. Much of the debate concerning the feasibility of hospital closure was, however, largely uninformed by research documenting the implementation of community care policies in practice and providing empirical evidence of their effects on the users and providers of the service. As discussed in chapter two of this volume, literature reviews in this area (Bassuk and Gerson, 1978; Braun et al.,1981; Thornicroft and Bebbington, 1989; and O'Driscoll, 1993) document the paucity of controlled outcome studies on the fate of long-stay patients being discharged from hospitals and highlight the urgent need for effective tracing systems and evaluation of aftercare for relocated patients.

As the closure of the North Wales Hospital was to be a flagship development in terms of hospital closure in Wales, providing a model for other districts to follow, the need to carry out a systematic evaluation of the resettlement of hospital residents was clearly important. To this end a joint proposal was developed between the relevant departments at University College North Wales and the Welsh Office, Department of Health, Health Authorities and Social Services Departments in Clwyd and Gwynedd. Within the context of the projected hospital closure, plans for the resettlement of long-stay patients from existing institutional care to a smaller scale domestic type of residential provision were prioritised. It was therefore decided that the evaluation of Clwyd's new mental health service should begin with the resettlement of long-stay patients. An independent research programme, the first of its kind in Wales dealing with psychiatric hospital closure, was seen as having a critical role to play in informing policy and practice concerning the implementation of the All Wales Strategy at both a local and national level.

It was therefore decided to fund a three year research project to evaluate the impact of the resettlement process on long-stay patients being discharged from the North Wales Hospital. This resulted in the establishment of the Health Services Research Unit (HSRU) in 1989 which initially constituted four full-time research workers with secretarial support. The HSRU was set up as a multi-disciplinary team linking the Departments of Psychology, the Centre for Social Policy Research and Development and the School of Accounting, Banking and Economics at the University College of North Wales. The team had its main base at the University and a second base at the hospital as the team were to work closely in liaison with psychiatrists and nursing staff involved in the resettlement programme. In April, 1989 work commenced on the first phase of the evaluation programme, focusing on the discharge of long-stay patients from the North Wales Hospital, Denbigh and an annexe at Pool Park Hospital, Ruthin.

As outlined in the original research proposal by Lowe, Grant, Morell, Alladin and Ellis (1988) the evaluation project was set up to monitor and evaluate the impact of the resettlement process on the lives of the individual patients as they were discharged from hospital. The study is therefore designed as a prospective longitudinal study which follows-up cohorts of patients as they are discharged from hospital, monitoring their level of functioning and quality of life in both the hospital and community care settings. The orientation of the study has as its prime focus the evaluation of the impact of resettlement on the well-being of patients leaving hospital. As such, a key component is the evaluation of the process from the perspective of the patients and its impact on their welfare. In addition to client outcomes the project also sets out to monitor changes in care practices as a result of the move to the community, evaluating changes in the quality of the care environments, care philosophy, management practices and staff attitudes. An economic analysis of the comparative costs of hospital and community-based care for the group of long-stay patients being resettled is also included as an important part of the evaluation project. The research programme therefore concerns itself with the process, outcome and cost consequences of the transfer of care for long-stay patients from hospital to community-based facilities.

The main aims of the study may be summarised as:

1. To provide objective evidence on whether care in the community does improve the quality of life and maintain the clinical well-being of long-stay patients discharged from hospital.
2. To assess the degree and direction of change in patient functioning related to the move from hospital to the community.
3. To evaluate and compare the process of care, including the care environments, care practices, assessment of need, and staff attitudes adopted by the hospital and community-based facilities.
4. To compare the economic costs of hospital care and care in the community and to compare costs across the different forms of community care.
5. To develop and refine existing research instruments to accomplish the objectives listed above.
6. To provide feedback to service providers that will inform policy and practice as the research proceeds.
7. To develop the research programme to include a comprehensive programme of evaluation which could be adapted for use with other client populations, and extended to address more specific evaluation questions as the research progresses.

The research protocol was specifically developed to include a comprehensive package of assessments to be undertaken with the patients, staff and agencies involved in the resettlement process. The protocol involves the collection of data from both clients and staff and includes structured and semi-structured interviews, self-completion questionnaires, rating scales, behavioural observation, documentary sources, participant observation. Full details of the research design, measures and the research cohort are to be found in chapter two.

During the course of the study, feedback from the project to planners and service providers was provided, generally in terms of average results, i.e. overall levels of functioning and quality of life for the group as a whole, not identifying specific individuals so as not to breach confidentiality. However, individual-based information was supplied in relation specific areas such as rehabilitation status as it was considered that such information was of direct clinical relevance and would therefore aid the staff in their development of individual care plans. While the HSRU team worked closely with the local agencies it was also important that the team should maintain its independent status and not become unduly involved in the planning and decision-making process. The focus of the team therefore remained the systematic evaluation of the resettlement process on the welfare of individual clients rather than its impact on the service system as a whole. Feedback was provided primarily through the dissemination of findings in reports and presentations targeted for policy makers, service providers, purchasers and care staff.

This publication brings together the findings from the first phase of the evaluation project, reporting on the first research cohort of long-stay patients resettled from the North Wales Hospital. Also included in this volume are details of the continuation of the evaluation programme to include the resettlement of remaining patients at the North Wales Hospital and the evaluation of the new community mental health teams being established in Clwyd and Gwynedd. The development work is being funded by the Department of Health and the Welsh Office and shows a change in the orientation of the research to address client groups in the community who are in receipt of the new community mental health services. The last three chapters of the book outline this second phase of the evaluation project and also include research studies being carried out at the Academic Sub-Department of Psychological Medicine, University of Wales College of Medicine. This work focuses on the development of community mental health teams in North Wales and reports on the introduction of user involvement strategies in the delivery of care.

References

Bassuk, E.L. and Gerson, S. (1978), *Deinstitutionalisation and Mental Health Services*. Scientific American, 238, 46-53.

Braun, P., Kochansky, G., Shapiro, R., Greenberg, S., Gudeman, J., Johnson, S., & Shore, M. (1981). 'Overview: Deinstitutionalization of psychiatric patients, a critical review of outcome studies', *American Journal of Psychiatry*, 138, 736-749.

Clwyd Health Authority (1987), 'Adult mental health strategy', *Consultative Document,* Clwyd Health Authority, Mold, North Wales.

Clwyd Health Authority (1991), *Clwyd County Plan for Mental Illness Services*. Clwyd Health Authority, Mold, North Wales

Lowe, C.F., Grant, G., Morrell, J.B., Alladin, W.J., Ellis, N.C. (1988), *Evaluation of the Mental Health Community Service in Clwyd: A research proposal*. University College of North Wales.

O'Driscoll, C. (1993), 'The TAPS Project 7: Mental hospital closure - A liturature review of outcome studies and evaluative techniques in J. Leff (ed). The TAPS Project: Evaluating Community Placement of Long-Stay Psychiatric Patients', *British Journal of Psychiatry*, 162 (suppl. 19), 7-17.

Thornicroft, G., and Bebbington, P. (1989), 'Deinstitutionalisation-from hospital closure to service development', *British Journal of Psychiatry,* 155, 739-753.

Welsh Office (1989), *Mental illness services: A strategy for Wales*, Welsh Office, Cardiff.

2 Evaluation of the North Wales Resettlement Programme: Methodology and cohort description

David A. Mitchell, Charles Crosby and Margaret M. Barry

Summary

This chapter provides a detailed description of the methodology used to evaluate the community resettlement of long-stay patients from the North Wales Hospital. The longitudinal design of the research is described in detail together with the selection, modification and development of the research instruments.

A comprehensive account is given of the characteristics of the research cohort participating in the study, constituting both old long-stay and new long-stay patients. Results of the hospital baseline assessments are presented together with a detailed examination of the psychometric properties of the measures used. The implications of the findings for the resettlement process are discussed.

Introduction

This chapter is intended primarily to provide a comprehensive description of the methodology and initial personal and psychiatric characteristics of the cohort involved in the evaluation of a community resettlement programme for residents of four wards in a large psychiatric hospital in North Wales. A detailed account of the research is of value for a number of reasons. First, in the absence of random sampling of both hospital and individuals involved, it cannot be known how representative the sample is of other psychiatric populations and institutions. Whether the findings of the present investigation should be generalized to other settings must therefore be judged on the similarity of the samples. The details presented in this chapter, along with the descriptions of the hospital and community environments and services provided elsewhere in this volume, will allow for a well informed judgement as to the applicability and relevance of the findings of the present resettlement programme to similar interventions in other places. Second, due to administrative fiat and clinical considerations, it was not possible to conduct a controlled investigation with random assignment of patients to treatment conditions. The validity of future conclusions regarding the effects of the resettlement programme is therefore dependent upon whether the alternative quasi-experimental design employed allows other plausible explanations of any pre- post-resettlement differences to be ruled out, or at least considered improbable. Finally, a description of the process involved and problems which arose in the design and implementation of the study should be of some heuristic value in that many of the difficulties encountered will not be unique to the present investigation. Indeed, many of the methodological concerns and difficulties which appeared are catholic to applied or field research in general and are particularly relevant for evaluation research.

Given that the policy of deinstitutionalisation has been actively pursued for more than three decades and has involved hundreds of thousands of individuals world-wide (see for example, Thornicroft & Bebbington, 1989), it is startling indeed that few systematic and rigourous evaluations of the process, and the consequences for those involved, have been undertaken. In describing and critically commenting on the first 20 years of deinstitutionalisation in the United States, Bassuk and Gerson (1978) noted that a major problem in determining the efficacy of reprovision of services in the community was the limited number of longitudinal studies of patients who had been discharged from large psychiatric hospitals. Reviewing the published research from the mid 1960s to the late 1970s, Braun, Kochansky, Shapiro, Greenberg, Gudemen, Johnson, and Shore (1981) identified only four experimental studies and one quasi-experimental study partially fulfilling criteria of methodological adequacy which attempted to evaluate alternatives to continued long-term hospitalisation. In summarizing their review, Braun et al. noted that, "few scientific studies are available with respect to deinstitutionalization of long-term patients in psychiatric hospitals ..." (p. 746) and concluded, "the failure to have evaluated adequately the effect of discharging hundreds of thousands of chronically ill patients from large public mental hospitals has been a major defect in the conduct of public policy" (p. 747). Notwithstanding this damning critique and recommendations for a more methodical approach to evaluation of all aspects of deinstitutionalisation, Braun's et al. counsel seems to have gone largely unheeded. In a recent selective, but what the author considered representative, review of the literature on mental hospital closure in the UK, the USA, and Italy, O'Driscoll (1993) stated that, "...much of the literature on deinstitutionalisation remains anecdotal or polemical, and there is a relative dearth of well constructed outcome studies to support or refute the validity of current policies" (p. 7). From the several hundred papers screened, O'Driscoll did not identify one which prospectively assessed the effects of closure of a mental hospital for the entire long-stay population. It seems that the policy of closing large mental hospitals and relocating long-stay patients in the community has been driven more by ideology than results of sound empirical research.

The comprehensive reviews by Braun et al. (1981) and O'Driscoll (1993) of studies of resettlement of long-stay psychiatric patients highlight a number of methodological inadequacies which preclude confident conclusions regarding the efficacy of alternatives to continued long-term hospitalisation. Some of the more pervasive deficiencies include; the use of a retrospective design, biased selection and uninformative sociodemographic and clinical description of patients, no pre-resettlement assessment, absent or incommensurable comparison group, the use of assessment procedures of unknown or questionable validity and reliability, inadequate and limited number of outcome criteria, and insufficient length of follow-up. These design and procedural inadequacies may, in isolation or in combination, seriously compromise various aspects of the validity of an investigation.

There are numerous potential confounding variables in any research, whether experimental or quasi-experimental, which may influence results and lead to misleading and invalid conclusions. Due to space limitations only those which are more problematic for evaluation research will be briefly discussed (for a comprehensive discussion see Cook and Campbell, 1979). Internal validity refers to the extent to which potentially confounding variables and alternative explanations for any observed 'effect' can be considered improbable. In the absence of random selection of subjects and assignment to treatment conditions, one of the major threats to the validity of an experiment is selection. A confound of selection can occur if comparisons are made between treated and non-treated groups when there are systematic differences in group composition. The possibility of a selection bias is especially probable if already formed or naturally occurring groups are used. Unless it can be demonstrated that the groups were equivalent on the measures of interest before the intervention, it cannot be known for certain if differences found after the manipulation are the result of the treatment or due to pre-existing differences. In addition, given that evaluation research usually entails a longitudinal design, i.e., at least two assessments spaced over a relatively long time, it is especially prone to a number of other confounding variables; maturation, history, testing, and instrumentation. The threat of maturation refers to systematic changes, physical or psychological, which occur within subjects over time irrespective of any treatment implementation (e.g., growing older). There can also be numerous extraneous events which occur over the course of the study that may affect the outcome. Such 'historical events' may be local (e.g., introduction of a new drug which coincides with an evaluation of the psychological effects of a resettlement programme) or more general (e.g., while evaluating the effects of a resettlement programme on quality of life, legislation is introduced to increase benefits paid to psychiatric patients). The threats of maturation and history become increasingly probable with longer pre-post-treatment measurement intervals. With repeated assessments there also exists the possible confound of testing effects. These are changes that occur which are the result of the measurement process itself. Having gained familiarity with the assessment procedure and the instruments used, subjects may formulate their own ideas about the purposes of the study and modify subsequent responses accordingly. If the assessment procedure involves human observers, the effects of being involved in the measurement process are not restricted only to the subjects of a study; with repeated use of a measurement instrument or procedure, observers may become more proficient in administering tests or more or less observant as the study progresses.

External validity, refers to the extent to which results of a study can be generalized to other persons, settings, and times. Although the immediate concern of evaluation research is to determine how successful a particular social or treatment programme is with a particular sample of individuals in a particular setting, the findings are often used to make an informed decision about the extension of the intervention to an overall population and/or other settings. Whether such generalizations are valid is dependent upon how well the initial sample accurately represents the population of interest. The method most often employed to achieve the goal of representativeness is random sampling of the population. However, in applied and evaluation research it is often difficult to accurately enumerate the population or the sample is specified in advance by policy makers or programme administrators.

Statistical validity, in a restricted sense, refers to the reliability of measures. Although there are different types, reliability refers to the reproducibility of measures. In order to produce useful data and have confidence in results it is essential the instruments employed consistently measure the concepts of interest. It is especially important to establish the reliability of measures which involve ratings done by human observers.

Construct validity is how well a particular measure accurately represents or reflects the theoretical construct of interest. Reliability and construct validity are related in that a measure must be reliable for it to be valid. As with internal and statistical validity there are several possible threats to construct validity.

Two of these are; 1) ambiguous or vague definitions of the relevant constructs; and, 2) the use of only one measure to represent the construct of interest (Cook & Campbell, 1979). The former threat is of particular significance for evaluation studies since it is often difficult to obtain precise specification of intended outcomes. In relation to rehabilitation programmes for psychiatric patients the general goals may be couched in terms such as 'to improve quality of life', 'to enhance social functioning', or 'to increase self-reliance'. Clearly, intended outcomes stated in this manner are inadequately specified for objective measurement. Concepts like 'quality of life', 'social functioning', etc., must be precisely defined so they can be operationalized and agreement reached that the measures used are valid indices of the construct. It is also prudent to use more than one measure to represent each of the constructs of interest because any one measure may not capture all the dimensions of a construct or, contain dimensions which are irrelevant to the construct of interest; what Cook and Campbell (1979) refer to as "construct underrepresentation" and "surplus construct irrelevancies", respectively. Using more than one measure acknowledges the fact that all measures contain error or unwanted variance and can increase construct validity by a convergence of measures which operationalize the same construct.

To the authors' knowledge, the only published study of the effects of resettlement of long-stay psychiatric patients which overcomes many of the inadequacies of methodology associated with earlier research is an on-going investigation being conducted by the Team for the Assessment of Psychiatric Services (TAPS) in London (Leff, 1993). The TAPS Project employs a prospective, longitudinal, quasi-experimental design and involves all patients (N = 770) residing in two large psychiatric hospitals under the age of 65 who had been hospitalized for more than one year (O'Driscoll & Leff, 1993). In addition to a research design which controls for many threats to internal validity, the TAPS Project also includes a comprehensive array of measurements; basic demographic information, psychiatric history, present mental state, physical health status, basic living skills, social behaviour and networks, patient attitudes to service provision, and an environmental index designed to measure the degree of autonomy, choices, and amenities available.

Preliminary results of the TAPS Project are encouraging in a number of respects. Of the 278 patients discharged during the first three years of the closure of the two hospitals, only 39 were readmitted once or more during a one year follow-up; all of whom returned to either their original reprovision setting or some other form of community placement (Dayson, 1993). Also of note is that in contrast to reports from the USA which have linked mental hospital closure to increased crime and homelessness (Bachrach, 1982; Weller, 1989), only one of the 278 was imprisoned at follow-up and one was definitely homeless and three others probably homeless. In comparison with a matched control group of patients who remained in hospital, the patients who were resettled had more diverse social networks, were more satisfied with their current placement, were living in a less restrictive environment, and did not show significant deterioration in psychiatric state or physical health (Anderson, Dayson, Wills, Gooch, Margolius, O'Driscoll, & Leff, 1993).

Notwithstanding the promising results from the first three years of the TAPS Project, there are reasons to treat the findings with some circumspection. The primary concern is that these interim results are based on a subsample of the total population of patients and there was a strong selection bias operating. In comparison to those remaining in hospital, the patients who had been resettled were significantly younger, had not been in hospital for as long, were more likely to have a diagnosis other than schizophrenia, had fewer social problems, had more extensive social networks, and were less likely to want to remain in hospital (Jones, 1993). Given the higher level of social functioning and greater desire to leave hospital, it could be argued that the patients who have been placed in the community are those who would be most likely to benefit from resettlement. Whether reprovision of care will be as successful for the remaining patients who are socially less able and who may be more difficult to place and maintain effectively in the community awaits further investigation.

Planning for the evaluation of the North Wales resettlement programme (Lowe, Grant, Morell, Alladin, & Ellis, 1988) was initiated before details of the TAPS Project were published and therefore was designed to address the apparent inadequacies of the seemingly extemporaneous investigations of alternatives to continued long-term hospitalisation of psychiatric patients which had been conducted previously. In addition to the need for a research design which would eliminate or reduce the influence of extraneous or confounding variables and allow for confidence in the validity of future findings and conclusions, two other methodological aspects were given particular attention; the nature and range of measures to be employed and the psychometric properties of the assessment instruments. The rationale and details of the research design adopted will be discussed subsequently (see Methodology) but, in summary, it took the form of a prospective, longitudinal, quasi-experimental design with multiple pre- and post-resettlement assessments. In terms of outcome measures a multi-method, multidisciplinary approach was adopted. Although the effects of community resettlement on patient functioning must take priority, hospital closure and reprovision of care also have economic consequences and implications for staff which reverberate throughout the local mental health care system. The economic effects with the consequent resource implications, along with staff attitudes concerning reprovision of services and the changes in care environment and management practices which resettlement entails, feed back and influence quality of care and, ultimately, patient welfare. To assess these indirect effects, an economic analysis and measurements of staff attitudes and management practices were included in the evaluation. These aspects of the research are dealt with elsewhere in this volume.

Outcome measures employed to assess direct effects of community resettlement on patients fall into two general, inter-related categories; patient functioning and quality of life. The latter aspect of the evaulation was included since one of the most frequently cited justifications for hospital closure is improved quality of life (Jones, 1988). As used in the present investigation, the concept encompasses not only objective and subjective indices of quality of life but also measures of patient satisfaction with service delivery. Details of the evaluation of the resettlement process on residents' quality of life can be found in chapter 6 in this volume.

The instruments used to assess patient functioning were selected on the basis of the suggestions of Hall (1979) who outlined a number of basic requirements of patient assessment procedures; amongst others, the use of more than one scale or type of assessment method, the use of standard assessment methods, and procedures which have been shown to be reliable. An additional requirement stated by Hall was that 'the reliability of any assessment method should not be assumed, but should be positively demonstrated during the study which is reported' (p. 334). Although the majority of the assessment procedures selected have been widely used in the psychiatric and rehabilitation literature, the evidence regarding their psychometric properties is, for most, not extensive. Hence, considerable attention has been given to investigation of the basic psychometric properties of the instruments used in data collection.

From a review of the relevant literature, examination of the impact of resettlement in three domains of patient functioning were identified as of importance; psychiatric state, social/life skills, and physical health. Based on the retrospective reports available it is difficult to specify the precise relationship between these areas of functioning and community resettlement. However, one assumption underlying the deinstitutionalisation movement is that reprovision of services in the community can provide care in a less restrictive setting as efficacious as hospital treatment and without the deleterious effects of social impoverishment and dependency producing environments associated with large psychiatric hospitals. In effect, a conservative prediction would be that resettlement should result in general improvement of quality of life and positive changes in social and interpersonal behaviours without any deterioration in psychiatric state or physical health.

Careful delineation of psychiatric state is important for at least two reasons. First, although considerable caution is needed in drawing conclusions from the available literature, it is apparent from results of previous resettlement initiatives for long stay psychiatric patients that programmes that have attempted to provide alternatives to in-patient care have not always met with the degree of success originally envisaged (Avison and Speechley, 1987; Braun et al., 1981). It is difficult to ascertain from these reports the precise reasons why some programmes of deinstitutionalisation have met with limited success; other than the explicit or implicit assumption that lack of adequate community resources and support are the major factors contributing to the failure of resettlement initiatives. There can be no doubt that provision for continuing support and availability and continuity of required resources are the foundations for successful community placement. However, these cannot be the only determinants of 'success' since even within a 'resource-rich service einvironment' (Geller, Fisher, Simon, & Wirth-Cauchon, 1990, p. 991) there are those individuals who adjust and integrate into the community and those who do not and subsequently 'relapse' and are readmitted to hospital. In this regard, certain characteristics such as age, major medical illness, length of hospitalisation, number of previous hospitalisations, and type and severity of psychiatric illness have, by exclusion criteria or on the basis of outcome, been suggested as possible variables affecting community placement. Such gross distinctions are not necessarily the most important criteria determining outcome since even within relatively homogeneous groups of patients, in terms of age and/or diagnostic group, outcome can be quite varied (e.g., Soni, Soni, & Freeman, 1978). What may be more important is the interaction between particular psychiatric attributes or symptoms and treatment milieus. Hemsley (1978) noted a number of reports of deterioration in the behaviour of schizophrenics taking part in intensive rehabilitation and token economy programmes. Wing (1975), in reviewing his own and related work on the effects of hospital environments and rehabilitation programmes, concluded that negative symptoms in schizophrenia occur more frequently and more intensely in conditions of social poverty while positive symptoms are more frequent and intense in socially overstimulating environments. The adverse effects of increased environmental stimulation is not limited to hospitalised patients. For example, Goldberg, Schooler, Hogarty, and Roper (1977) found that out-patients who entered an intensive rehabilitation programme with low levels of symptomatology faired much better that those who initially exhibited a greater number of and more intense symptoms. Likewise, Vaughan and Leff (1976) reported an increased rate of relapse for schizophrenics discharged to homes where the patient had frequent contact with relatives who expressed a high degree of emotion. Such findings have implications for any programme of resettlement given the likely increase in environmental stimulation which would follow from community placement.

The foregoing remarks have been restricted to predictive benefits which may accrue from the careful delineation and monitoring of psychiatric symptomatology. A second application of such a policy which is directly related to the current research is the assessment of outcome per se. In particular, there are no generally accepted operational criteria used to define outcome (Avison and Speechley, 1987). Falloon (1984), in a survey of treatment outcome studies of schizophrenia, found that no single criterion of relapse was common to all outcome studies. He reported that relapse was operationalized as:

> Admission to a psychiatric hospital unit, increase of medication, worsening of florid symptoms of schizophrenia, worsening of any psychiatric symptoms, and threatened clinical exacerbations have all been variables considered under the rubric of relapse. (Falloon, 1984, p. 295)

This has important implications for any research programme attempting to evaluate the process of deinstitutionalisation since the success or failure of such a programme may depend upon which criteria are used to define 'relapse'. Readmission to hospital, although the most widely used criterion, is of limited value since behavioural disturbance is differentially tolerated by different treatment settings and/or communities and is affected by a wide variety of social factors not related to symptoms (Wing, 1968). The use of repeated and objective assessment of psychiatric symptoms which takes into account not only the number present but also the intensity and extent to which these interfere with social functioning is likely to provide a more adequate means of determining the effects of resettlement on psychiatric state. A necessary prerequisite for such a methodology is to establish a baseline from which any change that may occur can be measured. Indeed, this is especially important when the majority of patients involved have a diagnosis of schizophrenia since it has been found from longitudinal studies that as much as 50 percent of these patients do not attain a stable clinical remission (Bleuler, 1974; Ciompi, 1980). This means that a simple absent (remission)/present (relapse) dichotomy is not appropriate. Rather, what is required is to establish the extent and intensity of symptoms before resettlement with any changes subsequent to community placement being related to this pre-discharge baseline. One complicating factor involved with such a design is that symptoms may not be stable over time but fluctuate in frequency, duration, and intensity of expression. It is therefore imperative that repeated assessments are carried out.

Although the foregoing discussion has concentrated on assessment of psychiatric symptomatology, this should not be taken to mean that other indices of patient functioning were relegated to a lesser role. It is appreciated that resettlement of itself may have effects other than those manifested by changes in psychiatric state. For example, a move from the socially impoverished and dependency producing environment of the large psychiatric hospital to the potentially more socially rich and self-reliant environment of the community may invoke changes in patients which could not be assessed by examination of mental state alone, e.g., degree of interpersonal interaction, changes in self-care and basic living skills, etc. In addition, it is desirable that assessment of patient functioning does not rely on the psychiatric interview as the only source of information. The use of behavioural rating scales which are completed by care staff, who are in daily contact with patients, can provide valuable information about behaviours which are not directly assessed in the psychiatric interview and which may have important implications for and about community placement.

The possible effect of deinstitutionalisation on the physical health of long-stay patients has received little attention in previous research reports. This is surprising since early reports (Aldrich & Mendkoff, 1963; Jasnau, 1967) found increased mortality rates amongst older patients transferred from long-stay institutions. Although later studies (Chanfreau, Deadman, George, & Taylor, 1990; Gutmann & Herbert, 1976) failed to replicate these findings and, in fact, some authors have even reported positive effects on self-perceived health (Borup, Gallego, & Heffernan, 1980), the possible effects of resettlement on the physical health of long-stay patients should not be ignored. Careful monitoring of physical health would also seem essential since it has been reported that there is increased physical illness and unmet physical health needs in chronic psychiatric patients in community settings (Brugha, Wing, & Smith, 1989; Honig, Pop, Tan, Philipsen, & Romme, 1989).

Methodology

Design

Due to clinical and administrative constraints the use of a true experimental design (i.e., random assignment of subjects to treatment conditions) was not feasible. Fortunately, however, the way in which the resettlement programme was to be implemented allowed for the use of a quasi-experimental design which was deemed to be practicable and efficacious. The design adopted can best be described as an interrupted time series with replications, i.e., repeated pre- and post-resettlement assessments on groups of individuals being moved to the community at staged intervals. Adapting the format of Cook and Campbell (1979), the design may be represented schematically as;

Group 1 $O11$ $O12$ $O13$ $O14$ X $O15$ $O16$ $O17$ ... $O1n$

Group 2 $O21$ $O22$ $O23$ $O24$ $O25$ X $O26$ $O27$ ... $O2n$

Group 3 $O31$ $O32$ $O33$ $O34$ $O35$ $O36$ X $O37$ ... $O3n$

.
.
.

Group z $Oz1$ $Oz2$ X   ... Ozn

with Ozn being measurement points and X the 'treatment' or, in this case, community resettlement.

In terms of internal validity, an interrupted time series with replications is potentially a very strong design. One advantage is that comparisons can not only be made between treatment and control conditions within the same subjects over time, but also between groups of subjects throughout a similar time window (Judd, Smith, & Kidder, 1991). Treatment effects within each group can be estimated by comparing the differences between points immediately preceding and following treatment implementation with differences between adjacent pretests. If the former are large and the latter small, this would constitute good evidence for a treatment effect. Threats such as maturation, instrumentation, and testing, which may compromise internal validity, can be assessed by examining the trends in the data before, at, and after the treatment. In addition, because the groups receive the treatment at different times, comparisons can be made between treated and untreated subjects at the same time and thereby assess the plausibility of one other rival explanation, that of history, which might account for pre- post-treatment differences. The rationale for this is that both the treated and non-treated groups would be exposed to similar historical events which coincided with the introduction of the treatment and so effects which may result from such exposure should be apparent in the treated and comparison groups. The threat of history cannot be completely eliminated however since it could be argued that, given the absence of random assignment, the treated and non-treated subjects may be differentially sensitive to historical events. Nonetheless, with multiple replications, the plausibility of post-treatment changes being attributable to selection and/or selection-history interactions becomes less probable.

Given that random assignment of subjects to treatment conditions was not feasible, the design adopted capitalizes on the administrative/logistic constraints placed on the resettlement programme. In particular, patients were to be resettled depending upon the availability of appropriate community residences. This meant that groups of individuals would be placed in the community at different times. These stages or waves of resettlement would allow for replications of treatment implementation and also result in a residual pool of patients left in hospital which could be used as a non-equivalent comparison group. In addition, because the intended move from hospital based to community based provision of care was known long before the policy was to be implemented, the opportunity existed for conducting a number of pre-resettlement assessments. This raised the question of how often and how many assessments should be carried out to accurately reflect symptom oscillations. Given the absence of any a priori knowledge of the 'signal' parameters, it is difficult to specify the most appropriate sampling frequency in advance. There are however at least three factors which can aid in this decision.

Firstly, there is the clinical knowledge that once a patient has been 'stabilized' on a treatment regime, he or she, by definition, no longer exhibits the extremes of behavioural disturbance that led to intervention. This is not to say that all symptoms have been ameliorated but rather that, if still present, the intensity, duration, and/or frequency of symptom expression has been reduced. It does not seem unreasonable to assume that with continued hospitalisation and the consequent buffering effect of the hospital environment and opportunity for observation and changes in treatment strategy, control of symptoms will become ever more refined until a plateau is reached where no further improvement can be realized. If this reasoning is accepted, it follows that the number and frequency of sampling intervals needed to reflect symptom expression will be partially a function of the length of hospitalisation and hence fewer will be required to accurately characterize individuals who have been in hospital for longer periods of time. Second, a simple empirical approach can be adopted whereby if results are stable across two or three occasions spaced over a reasonable time window there would be little incremental value in continuing to repeat assessments. The third factor is simply practical in nature; the number of assessments is limited by available personnel and time. In practice, available resources is usually the limiting factor which forces a compromise between what the researcher would like to do and what is feasible.

With these considerations in mind, it was decided that a minimum of three assessments at approximately three month intervals would be carried out before community placement. In addition to these baseline measurements, each individual would be assessed one week prior to being resettled. The latter sampling point was added to ensure the last hospital based assessment was coeval with community placement. Given that the majority of the individuals in the sample had been hospitalized and had resided on the same ward for many years, the assessment one week prior to resettlement would also detect symptom exacerbation and behavioural deterioration which might be associated with the stress induced by the impending move to a new environment. For comparison purposes, individuals remaining in hospital after each wave of resettlement would continue to be monitored at appropriate intervals.

As with baseline assessments, determination of the most appropriate post-resettlement sampling frequency and period was problematic. Ideally, assessments should be conducted at the same interval used prior to community placement. However, because patients were to be dispersed in small groups to community residences throughout North Wales, logistic, budgetary, and personnel constraints placed severe restrictions on the number and frequency of post-resettlement assessments. Given these limitations, it was decided the follow-up period would be, initially, one year with three assessments being conducted; one at six weeks, one at six months, and one at the end of the first year.

Methods of assessment

Personal Data and History Form (PDHF). The PDHF allows a standardized means of collecting basic personal and demographic data (age, sex, place of birth, educational and employment history, etc.) and information regarding an individual's psychiatric history (number and duration of previous admissions, age of first psychiatric contact, diagnoses, etc.). Case-notes were perused to complete the PDHF.

Brief Psychiatric Rating Scale (BPRS). The Brief Psychiatric Rating Scale as originally described by Overall and Gorham (1962) consists of 16 symptom constructs which are rated on scales ranging from 1 ('not

18

present') to 7 ('extremely severe'). Experience in using the BPRS during the initial stages of baseline assessments, when ratings were done by consensus agreement between two raters, suggested two inadequacies with the original scale: 1) Agreement between raters in terms of severity of a particular symptom was difficult due to there being no guide-lines in the scale for deciding between, say, 'very mild' 'mild' or even 'moderate' degrees of symptomatology. 2) Assessment of symptoms of importance for manic disorders and indices of possible organic dysfunction were inadequately covered. In light of these observations, it was decided to adopt some of the modifications to the BPRS proposed by Lukoff, Liberman, & Nuechterlein (1986). In particular, Lukoff et al. provided explicit descriptions for the seven points for each of the symptoms. To compensate for what was felt to be inadequate symptom coverage, four additional scales (Elevated Mood, Motor Hyperactivity, Distractibility, and Disorientation) from Lukoff's et al. modifications were adopted along with one (Incomprehensible Speech) devised by the Health Services Research Unit (HSRU) team. This modified version of the BPRS, consisting of 21 symptom constructs each with explicit criteria for ratings of severity on a 7-point scale ranging from 0 ('not present') to 6 ('extremely severe'), was subsequently adopted with independent ratings being made by two observers to allow for assessment of inter-rater reliability.

Krawiecka Rating Scale (KRS). The Krawiecka Rating Scale (Krawiecka, Goldberg, & Vaughan, 1977) consists of eight 5-point scales (0 'absent' to 4 'severe') designed to provide a clinical assessment of chronic psychotic patients. Unlike the original version of the BPRS, the KRS has explicit criteria for assigning subjects to each of the five points on the eight scales. Although there is considerable overlap in the symptom constructs covered by the BPRS and the KRS, it has been suggested that the KRS is more sensitive to change (Krawiecka et al., 1977). As with the BPRS, ratings by consensus were initially conducted in order for areas of disagreement and differences in interpretation to be revealed. In general, obtaining inter-rater agreement proved satisfactory. The one rating which did present some difficulty in obtaining a consensus was that for the symptom of Flattened Affect. The equivalent items (Blunted Affect and Emotional Withdrawal) on the BPRS also presented problems in arriving at agreement between raters. This is not too surprising however given the rather vague and ill-defined nature of these items on both the BPRS and KRS, e.g., 'reduced emotional tone' 'failing to be in emotional contact' 'impairment in the range of available emotional responses'. In fact, of the eight ratings on the KRS, Krawiecka et al. (1977) reported Flattened Affect to have the lowest inter-rater agreement in two reliability studies. Given this apparent deficiency with the BPRS and KRS it was decided to operationalise the constructs of Blunted-Flattened Affect by including an additional scale in the assessment procedure; one of the global measures from Andreasen's (1982) Scale for the Assessment of Negative Symptoms.

19

Scale for the Assessment of Negative Symptoms-Affective Flattening (SANS-AF). The Scale for Assessment of Negative Symptoms (SANS) was developed by Andreasen and co-workers (Andreasen, 1982; Andreasen & Olsen, 1982) in order to provide clearly defined, operational criteria for the assessment of the 'negative' symptoms of schizophrenia. In it's original form, the SANS contains five global symptom complexes (alogia, affective flattening, avolition-apathy, anhedonia-asociality, and attentional impairment) each of which is defined by observable behavioural components that are rated on a six-point scale (0 'not present' to 5 'severe'); all of which have been shown to allow for high inter-rater reliability (Andreasen, 1982). Of the five global measures, the one of interest for present purposes is that of Affective Flattening. This particular symptom complex was originally defined by Andreasen (1982) as being composed of nine ratings based on behaviour during an interview. Consideration of these nine items led the present investigators to drop three (Inappropriate Affect, Subjective Rating of Affective Flattening and a Global Rating) because they either seemed inappropriate or, due to the criteria used, would present similar difficulties to those which the SANS was introduced to alleviate, i.e., highly subjective criteria. To distinguish it from the original, this will be referred to as the SANS-AF (Affective Flattening). It should be noted that the SANS was incorporated part-way through the initial baseline assessments and therefore analyses involving this instrument involved a reduced sample size.

Present State Examination (PSE). The PSE (Wing, Cooper, & Sartorius, 1974) is a well-established, standardized, semi-structured interview schedule which allows for ratings of individuals on the major symptoms of psychiatric disorders over the previous month. Although the PSE was not developed specifically for diagnostic purposes but rather to provide a clear, precise, and reliable description of clinical phenomena (Wing, 1983), it's comprehensive coverage of psychiatric symptomatology does allow for the generation of diagnoses using different nosological systems. In addition, when used in conjunction with an associated computer program, CATEGO, patients may be described in terms of symptom profiles, syndromes, a CATEGO class (i.e., classification based on CATEGO-specific criteria; as opposed to a clinical diagnosis), and a tentative ICD-9 diagnosis. All PSE interviews were conducted by a senior registrar from NWH, Dr Carl Littlejohns, who had formal training in its use.

OPCRIT. The OPCRIT (McGuffin, Farmer, & Harvey, 1991) is a 74-item computer-evaluated questionnaire which is completed by examination of case-notes. It allows for the allocation of individuals to diagnostic categories on the basis of differing criteria employed by various nosological systems. It should be noted that unlike the PSE, which as used in the present research rated only those symptoms which occurred during the previous month, ratings for the OPCRIT were based on all available historical information, i.e., life-time diagnoses. The OPCRIT was completed by a senior registrar from NWH, Dr Frederick Harrocks.

Rehabilitation Scale of Hall and Baker (REHAB). The REHAB (Baker and Hall, 1983) is a standardized scale to assess the rehabilitation status of psychiatric patients and has received wide currency in the literature. Ratings are carried out by care staff on the basis of the patient's behaviour over the previous week. The scale is divided into two parts; ratings for frequency of seven Deviant Behaviours (e.g., incontinence, violence, self-injury) and on a 10-point analogue scale for 16 General Behaviours (e.g., social interactions, self-care, community skills). To allow for assessment of inter-rater reliability, each patient was rated by two members of care staff independently. All staff members who completed ratings were, individually, given a description of the REHAB and instructed in its use by the members of the HSRU team. In addition, one member of the research team was present while staff completed the ratings to clarify any subsequent difficulties with interpretation of items.

Physical Health Index (PHI). The PHI (O'Driscoll, 1985) is intended to give an approximation of the level of physical disability and care needs of psychiatric patients. Functioning in seven bodily systems (cardiovascular, respiratory, gastrointestinal, urogenital, locomotor, nervous, and endocrine/metabolic) is evaluated by obtaining information from case-notes and nursing staff. Each system is evaluated for the presence of any problems and, if present, rated for degree of impairment of the individual's physical functioning and the level of medical/nursing care received. Five 'critical' disabilities (incontinence, impaired mobility, blindness, deafness, and dyskinesias) are also rated for presence/absence. The PHI was completed by the senior registrars, Drs Horrocks and Littlejohns.

General procedure

For the initial baseline assessment, ratings of psychiatric symptomatology were conducted during two separate interviews: one by members of the HSRU team, who completed the Brief Psychiatric Rating Scale and the Krawiecka Rating Scale, and one by a senior registrar based at North Wales Hospital, Denbigh who administered the Present State Examination. Although an attempt was made to co-ordinate the HSRU team's interview with that of the senior registrar conducting the PSE, due to clinical commitments of the latter, this was not always possible.

Given that the reliability of any psychiatric rating scale is dependent not only on the explicitness and clarity of the criteria used for rating a particular symptom, but also consistency between raters in areas of inquiry and the means by which information is elicited (Beck, Ward, Mendelson,

Mock, & Erbaugh, 1962), it was thought desirable to develop a standard interview for use by the HSRU team. Items included in the schedule were developed, or chosen from other published interviews, primarily the PSE and BPRS interview schedule suggested by Lukoff et al. (1986), to compliment the symptoms which were to be rated on the BPRS and KRS. The interview procedure was developed from a pilot study and resulted in a 45 item schedule which takes approximately 20-30 minutes to complete and allows for ratings on the BPRS and KRS to be carried out.

One week prior to ratings on the REHAB, key workers for each patient were contacted and asked if they would be willing to participate. A brief description of the research project was given along with an introduction to the scale they would be required to complete one week hence. Having made this arrangement, patients were then scheduled to be interviewed by members of the HSRU team during the appointed week. Where possible, interviews were conducted on the same day the REHAB was completed.

Each patient was approached individually by members of the HSRU team and, having been given a description of the project, was asked if he or she would participate in the research. If so, the patient was asked to sign an informed consent form. The interview itself took approximately one hour to complete and included all questions from the psychiatric interview schedule and Quality of Life Questionnaire. Ratings on the BPRS, KRS, and SANS-AF were completed immediately after each interview.

The same general procedure employed during initial baseline assessments was adopted for all subsequent assessment points (see below); the exceptions being the PSE and the OPCRIT which were administered/completed at the first assessment only.

Data reduction and analyses

Subjects were assigned an identification number prior to data being entered on a Macintosh SE/30 computer. Separate databases were created for each measurement instrument using FoxBase+ (Fox Software, 1988). All data were subsequently transferred to the UCNW Vax mainframe for statistical analyses. The SPSS-x (SPSS Inc., 1988) package was used for all analyses.

Data reduction

In most analyses of the BPRS, KRS, SANS-AF, and REHAB items, mean scores of two raters were used. For BPRS and KRS data collected during the initial stages of baseline assessments, ratings arrived at by consensus were taken as a 'mean' rating.

For the BPRS, KRS, and REHAB the number of items was further reduced by computing composite scores. Based on the results of a factor analysis of the BPRS from a sample of 3596 subjects, Overall and Gorham

(1976) suggest the use of five 'factor' scores plus a total score, i.e., the sum of all items. Table 2.1 presents the item composition of each factor score. Item composition for the factors Anergia and Activation differ from that of Overall and Gorham in that one item from each was dropped (Disorientation and Motor Hyperactivity, respectively).

Table 2.1
Item composition of the five factors used for analysis of the BPRS

i	*Anxiety- Depression*	Somatic Concern
		Anxiety
		Guilt Feelings
		Depressive Moods
ii	*Anergia*	Emotional Withdrawal
		Motor Retardation
		Blunted Affect
iii	*Thought Disturbance*	Conceptual Disorganisation
		Grandiosity
		Hallucinatory Behaviour
		Unusal Thought Content
iv	*Activation*	Tension
		Mannerisms and Posturing
v	*Hostile-Suspiciousness*	Hostility
		Suspiciousness
		Uncooperative

Factor Score - Sum of composite items/Number of composite items

This was done because the version of the BPRS used by Overall and Gorham contained 18 items, as opposed to the original 16-item version initially used in the present evaluation. Omitting these two items allowed for calculation of all five factor scores for the total sample. In the first instance, it is these scores which were analysed. Where significant effects were found, each individual item contributing to a particular factor score was subsequently analysed to determine the individual item(s) of significance. The two items omitted from the factor scores and the additional items (Elevated Mood, Distractability, Incomprehensible Speech) in the 21-item version of the BPRS subsequently adopted were analysed individually.

Four composite scores were also computed for the KRS; Anxious-Depressed (mean of ratings for anxiety and depression), Thought Disorder (mean of ratings for hallucinations, delusions, and incoherent speech), Poverty (mean of ratings for poverty of speech, flattened affect, and motor retardation), and a total score.

Baker and Hall (1983) provide a means of computing additive scales for the General Behaviour items of the REHAB. From a factor analysis of scores from a sample of 508 long stay patients, they reported five factors. These, along with items which loaded on each, are presented in Table 2.2.

Baker and Hall suggest that sub-scale scores may be computed by simply summing the relevant items for each factor. A total score is also calculated by summing all items from the General Behaviour items. As with analysis of the BPRS, initial analyses used the 'factor' scores with subsequent analysis of individual items when a significant effect was found.

Table 2.2

Item composition of the five factors used for analysis of the REHAB

i	Social Activity	Mixing on Ward
		Mixing off Ward
		Use of Spare Time
		Level of Activity
		Amount of Speech
		Imitation of Speech
ii	Speech Disturbance	Sense of Speech
		Clarity of Speech
iii	Self Care	Table Manners
		Washing Self
		Dressing Self
		Looking after Possessions
		Amount of Prompting
iv	Community Skills	Use of Money
		Use of Public Facilities
v	Speech Skills	Amount of Speech
		Initiation of Speech

Factor Score = Sum of Composite Items

Total General Behaviour = I + II + III + IV + Overall Rating

Analyses involving the SANS-AF were carried out on the total score, i.e, the sum of all six items.

Analyses

Inter-rater reliability. Inter-rater reliability was assessed using the Kappa family of statistics; for nominal data Cohen's Kappa (K) and, for quantitative data, intraclass correlation coefficients (ICC). These statistics are preferable to more commonly used measures of agreement such as per cent agreement, product moment correlations, and rank order correlations (Bartko, 1976; Bartko and Carpenter, 1976). For nominal data, Cohen's K corrects for chance agreements; which can be numerous if few categories are used by raters or the base rate of the behaviour/construct in the sample under investigation is either very low or very high. Values of K range from 1.0 for perfect agreement through 0 for chance agreement to negative values for less than chance. Values greater than 0.75 are generally taken to indicate excellent agreement beyond chance, values below 0.40 representing poor agreement beyond chance, with values between representing fair to good agreement beyond chance (Fleiss, 1981).

Product moment and rank order correlations may also be spuriously high inter-rater reliability estimates. This can occur when one rater has an additive or multiplicative bias in relation to another rater, i.e., as long as raters co-vary consistently, reliability, as inferred from these statistics, will appear high irrespective of the actual level of agreement. The ICC, by comparing the variance within to that between a set of measurements, is not subject to this spurious inflation of reliability estimates. Another distinct advantage of the ICC, and K, is that they can be tested for statistical significance. Overall, the assessment of inter-rater agreement has been more rigourous than is usually the case.

Results

Demographic and clinical characteristics

Table 2.3 presents personal and psychiatric history data for the total sample.

Table 2.3
Demographic and clinical characteristics for the total sample

Sample		N	65	
Age (years)		Mean	55.1	
		SD	15.4	
		Range	26.5 - 85.7	
Sex	Males	N	55	
	Females		10	
Ever married		N	5	
Have/Had children		N	3	
Status	Informal	N	59	
	Section		6	
Diagnosis from Case Notes	Schiz	N	50	(76.9%)
	Other		11	(16.9%)
	Not known		4	(6.1%)
Length of present stay (years)		Mean	21.1	
		SD	16.9	
		Range	.4 - 61.6	
Age of first psychiatric contact		Mean	24.2	
		SD	8.5	
		Range	12 - 57	
Total years hospitalised		Mean	24.8	
		SD	16	
		Range	.7 - 61.6	
Number of admissions		Mean	4.2	
		Range	1 - 20	
Average durations of stay per admission (years)		Mean	17.0	
		SD	17.0	
		Range	.1 - 60.6	
Positive family history		N	18	(27.7%)

With the exception of five, for whom place of birth could not be established with certainty, all individuals had been born in the United Kingdom; 42 in Wales, 15 in England, and three in Scotland. Of those for whom an employment history could be unequivocally determined, 12 had never worked, 31 had been employed in unskilled and eight in skilled manual jobs, three had done some form of clerical work, and two had been in the Services. It is noteworthy that only five of the 65 (approximately 8%) were, or had been, married with three (4.6%) having children; these proportions are considerably smaller than would be expected given the age range of the sample.

From medical records, 77% of the sample had a primary clinical diagnosis of some type of schizophrenia (including schizo-affective). The remaining 17% for whom a diagnosis could be ascertained were rather heterogeneous and included two each of mental deficiency and epilepsy, and one each of unipolar depression, manic-depressive illness, congenital neurosyphilis, acute psychosis, brain damage, asocial behaviour, and 'not psychiatrically ill'. A clinical diagnosis could not be found in the case-notes for four individuals.

Table 2.4 presents the percentages of patients who met diagnostic criteria for 'schizophrenia' using the nosological systems included in the OPCRIT and the percentages given an ICD-9 diagnosis of schizophrenia and assigned to class S+ on the basis of PSE data as analysed by CATEGO. As can be seen from this table, the life-time diagnoses of the various diagnostic systems included in the OPCRIT support the clinical diagnosis of schizophrenia. Although there is an overall effect between diagnostic systems for differences in the proportions of patients classified as schizophrenic (Cochran's Q = 13.47, p < .05), paired comparisons (using McNemar's test) of the various diagnostic systems and clinical diagnosis were all non-significant.

Table 2.4
Percentages of sample meeting diagnostic criteria for schizophrenia using various classification systems

Diagnosis from OPCRIT	DSM III	74.6	(59)
	DSM III-R	69.5	(59)
	RDC	69.5	(59)
	Feighner	72.9	(59)
	Carpenter Flexible System	83.0	(59)
	Taylor and Abrams	72.9	(59)
	Schneiderian FRSs	37.3	(59)
Diagnosis and Classification from PSE Data	ICD-9	38.2	(55)
	Catego Class S+*	25.5	(55)

* Index of Definition greater than or equal to 5

In contrast to the results from the OPCRIT, which uses all available data from the psychiatric history, the PSE, as used in the present study, is based only on the psychiatric state of the individual over the previous month. As can be seen from Table 2.4, when diagnosis and classification are based on present state only, the proportion of individuals diagnosed as schizophrenic, or exhibiting what are considered by some (e.g., Wing et al., 1974) to be the cardinal features of schizophrenia (CATEGO class S), is reduced markedly. The differences in the proportion of subjects assigned an ICD-9 diagnosis of schizophrenia and class S are both significantly different from the proportion having a clinical diagnosis of schizophrenia ($x2 = 18.89$ and 25.71, respectively, $p < .000$). As might be expected, the proportions of individuals assigned to class S by CATEGO are very similar to the proportions who have exhibited Schneiderian first rank symptoms (FRS) at some time during their psychiatric history; CATEGO relies heavily on the presence of FRSs for a classification of schizophrenia (class S). If the classes of 'Other Psychosis' (O+ and O?) and 'Paranoid' (P+ and P?) are also considered to represent what other classification systems would consider 'schizophrenia', the per cent of patients so classified by CATEGO would rise to 56.4, a proportion more in line with that of the diagnostic systems of the OPCRIT.

Five of the sample were not prescribed any medication or were taking medicine for a physical complaint only. Of the remaining 60, 59 or approximately 90% of the total sample were receiving at least one form of psychotropic drug; one individual was taking an anticonvulsant only.

Table 2.5
Demographic and clinical characteristics for
new and old-long stay patients (N=65)

		NLS		OLS	
N		18		46	
Age (yrs)	Mean	40.9		60.9	
	SD	11.5		13.1	
Sex	Males	13		41	
	Females	5		5	
Ever married	N	4		1	
Have/had children	N	3		1	
Clinical Diagnosis	Schizophrenia	13	(72.2%)	37	(80.4%)
	Other	5	(27.8%)	6	(13.0%)
	Not known			3	(6.5%)
Length of present stay (yrs)	Mean	2.4		28.6	
	SD	1.7		14.2	
	Range	.5 - 5.7		7.1 - 61.6	
Age of first psychiatric	Mean	23.7		24.4	
contact	SD	6.3		9.1	
	Range	17 - 40		12 - 57	
Total years hospitalised	Mean	7.7		31.3	
	SD	11.2		12.4	
Number of admissions	Mean	8.3		2.67	
	Range	1 - 20		1 - 14	
Average duration of stay per	Mean	2.8		22.0	
admission (yrs)	SD	5.93		16.6	

Thirty-five were on a depot preparation with the remaining 24 receiving an oral antipsychotic. Twenty-six of the 35 receiving injections were also taking daily doses of an oral antipsychotic. Antiparkinsonians were prescribed for 41. Six of those receiving an antipsychotic were also prescribed an anticonvulsant.

The relatively high proportion (28%) of the sample with a relative who had some form of psychiatric disorder is notable; even more so since it would not be unreasonable to assume that this figure is probably an under-estimate of the actual proportion given that these data were obtained from case-notes. Of the 18 affected relatives, 13 were from the patient's immediate family (i.e., mother, father, sister, or brother). Of the 13, seven had been diagnosed as either schizophrenic or depressive; a diagnostic category was not recorded for the others. Of the remaining five patients, one had a grandfather who had been diagnosed schizophrenic and two had a grandfather, one a cousin, and one an aunt who had an unspecified psychiatric or 'nervous' disorder.

In general, these results indicate a sample comprised largely of individuals who may be considered 'chronic' in terms of their psychiatric history. It also seems that the sample may be divided into two sub-groups; one of older individuals who have been in hospital for a large proportion of their lives and with few admissions; and, a younger group which is characterised by frequent, relatively short stays in hospital. It may be that these two groups represent what have been termed 'old' and 'new' long stay patients, respectively (Wing, 1971). In fact, on inspection of the distribution of values for the present length of hospitalisation, the sample could be conveniently divided into two groups; those whose current period in hospital was less than seven years and those who had been in hospital for more than seven years.

Four individuals in the former group did not strictly meet the criteria normally used to define new long stay patients (e.g., Wykes, 1982) since they had been hospitalized for less than one year. However, three had been in hospital longer than six months and all had a history not dissimilar to those who had been in hospital one year to seven years, i.e., numerous, relatively short previous admissions. The one remaining individual had been hospitalized less than six months and had no known previous admissions and was therefore not included in either group. Table 2.5 summarizes demographic and psychiatric history profiles for, what will subsequently be referred to as, the old long stay (OLS) and new long stay (NLS) groups.

Psychiatric assessment

Table 2.6 presents intra-class correlation coefficients (ICC) and associated F-values for all symptom ratings on the BPRS, KRS, and SANS-AF obtained during initial baseline assessment. All coefficients are significant at the .01 level or greater.

As would be expected, reliabilities for the composite scores for the three scales were generally better than those for individual items; .80, .75, .83, .67, .80, and .81 for the BPRS factors of Anxiety-Depression, Anergia,

Thought Disturbance, Activation, Hostile-Suspiciousness, and Total BPRS, respectively; .37, .86, .78, and .69 for the KRS composite scores of Anxious-Depressed, Thought Disorder, Poverty, and Total, respectively; and, .77 for the Total SANS-AF. Overall, the ICCs presented in Table 2.6 are very encouraging with some representing what must be considered exceptionally good agreement between raters, i.e., .90, .90, .91 for Somatic Concern, Grandiosity, and Hallucinations of the BPRS, respectively, .99 for Hallucinations on the KRS, and .91 for amount of Eye Contact on the SANS-AF. What this means is that less than, approximately, 10% of the variance (i.e., 1-ICC) is due to error or disagreement between raters. Of the remaining 18 ICCs for the scales of the BPRS, 16 can be considered to represent good to very good inter-rater agreement.

Table 2.6
ICCs for symptom rating on BPRS, KRS, and SANS-AF

	Symptom	ICC	F-Value
BPRS	Somatic Concern	.90	19.11
	Anxiety	.70	5.69
	Despressive Mood	.66	4.90
	Guilt Feelings	.65	4.70
	Hostility	.72	6.21
	Suspiciousness	.70	5.68
	Unusual Thought Content	.74	6.76
	Grandiosity	.90	20.11
	Hallucinations	.91	22.05
	Elevated Mood	.78	8.12
	Disorientation	.75	7.10
	Conceptual Disorganisation	.47	2.79
	Incomprehensible Speech	.78	7.94
	Motor Hyperactivity	.61	4.16
	Motor Retardation	.78	8.18
	Blunted Affect	.66	4.90
	Tension	.63	4.39
	Mannerisms and Posturing	.63	4.41
	Uncooperativeness	.81	9.24
	Emotional Withdrawal	.71	5.92
	Distractability	.68	5.20
KRS	Depressed	.58	3.72
	Anxious	.43	2.48
	Delusions	.82	10.36
	Hallucinations	.99	208.23
	Incoherence	.54	3.34
	Poverty of Speech	.80	8.79
	Flattened Affect	.65	4.67
	Psychomotor Retardation	.56	3.51
SANS-AF	Facial Expression	.62	4.32
	Spontaneous Movements	.63	4.42
	Expressive Gestures	.77	7.69
	Eye Contact	.91	20.36
	Affective Responsivity	.53	3.30
	Vocal Inflections	.70	5.66

Likewise, six of the remaining seven ratings on the KRS and four of the remaining five SANS-AF ratings can be considered as representing good to very good agreement.

Subsequent to the first round of assessments, work continued on the rating scales to improve their reliability even further with special attention being given to those for which inter-rater agreement was relatively low. Calculation of ICCs for the first 28 and 34 subjects' data collected during the first and second retest, respectively, revealed a general improvement in inter-rater agreement. For example, ICCs for three of the factor scores (Anxiety-Depression, Thought Disturbance, and Hostile-Suspiciousness) and Total score for the BPRS exceeded .9 for the first retest. The ICC for Activation remained unchanged while that for Anergia showed a slight decrease (.67). A similar improvement was found for the KRS composite scores; .71, .92, .67, and .78 for Anxious-Depressed, Thought Disorder, Poverty, and Total score, respectively. The ICC for the Total SANS-AF score was also somewhat higher (.81) than found for ratings at initial baseline assessment and this improvement was maintained for the second retest (ICC = .79). Mean ICCs for the BPRS and KRS factor scores were .78 and .72, respectively, for the second retest.

In general, there are few published findings with which the above results can be compared. In spite of the BPRS being one of the most widely used clinical rating instruments (Alpert, 1985), there are few published studies which have reported inter-rater reliability estimates for individual symptom ratings and factor scores. In their original publication, Overall and Gorham (1962) reported reliability coefficients ranging from .87, for Guilt Feelings and Hallucinations, to .56, for Tension. Of the 16 ratings common to Overall and Gorham's original scale and those included in the version of the BPRS used in the present research, seven of the scales in the present study had higher and eight had lower reliability coefficients (the coefficients for Blunted Affect were equivalent) than those reported by Overall and Gorham. The method of computing inter-rater reliability (ICC) in the present study was, however, much more stringent than that of Overall and Gorham who used product-moment correlations for reliability estimates. It will be recalled that product-moment correlations are likely to be over-estimates of reliability. In general, it would therefore seem that inter-rater reliability in the present research is as good, if not better, than that reported by Overall and Gorham. The only published study which the authors are aware of that has used ICCs as estimates of inter-rater reliability for individual items and factor scores for the BPRS is that of Lukoff et al. (1986). Unfortunately, they did not report coefficients for all the symptom ratings. Lukoff et al. reported ICCs of .93, .97, .73, .90, and .89 for Unusual Thought Content, Hallucinations, Conceptual Disorganization, Depression, and Hostility, respectively. Although these coefficients are higher than those found in the present investigation (see Table 2.6), these are not directly comparable since the values reported by Lukoff et al. are median coefficients of seven raters.

There are even fewer published studies which have reported on the reliability of the KRS. In fact, the only study that the authors are aware that has assessed inter-rater reliability of individual symptom ratings for the KRS is that of Krawiecka et al. (1977). These authors reported coefficients ranging from .87, for ratings of Depressed, to .58, for ratings of Flattened, Incongruous Affect. Once again, however, these coefficients are not directly comparable to those presented here since Krawiecka et al. used Kendall's Coefficient of Concordance for estimating reliability. Their coefficients were in effect the average degree of association between five rater's scores. It is not too surprising therefore that the ICCs found for the ratings in the present investigation are somewhat lower, i.e., more stringent criteria and actual agreement between two raters.

Unlike the situation for the BPRS and KRS, there are published reports which have assessed inter-rater reliability of the SANS-AF which are directly comparable to the present findings. For example, Andreasen (1982) reported ICCs ranging from .70 to .91 for the six SANS-AF items used here. With the exception of one, Eye Contact, Andreasen's reliability estimates are higher than those listed in Table 2.6. It is important to note however that the raters in Andreasen's study used the full version of the SANS and completed the ratings after reviewing ward records and nursing notes concerning psychiatric history and behaviour and discussing the patient's behaviour directly with nursing personnel. These additional data may have influenced the ratings of behaviour observed during the interview. In fact, the inter-rater reliability estimates were based on a sub-sample of a larger sample. In a subsequent report which included all subjects, Andreasen and Akiskal (1983) report ICCs which are more in line with those found in the present investigation; .73, .71, .57, .79, .36, and .51 for Unchanging Facial Expression, Decreased Spontaneous Movements, Paucity of Expressive Gestures, Poor Eye Contact, Affective Nonresponsivity, and Lack of Vocal Inflections, respectively. By reference to Table 2.6, it can be seen that the ICCs for four of the six scales are higher than those reported by Andreasen and Akiskal.

A second means of assessing the reliability of a measurement instrument is test-retest reliability. Notwithstanding the argument that test-retest is not an appropriate measure of reliability for psychiatric rating scales (i.e., symptom expression fluctuates over time), correlations between assessment points were calculated for two reasons. First, the majority of the sample had been in hospital for a prolonged period and thus, although still exhibiting symptoms, should have been stabilized on the most appropriate treatment regime. Second, one item from the REHAB requires the rater to assess whether, over the past week, the patients behaviour, in general, is worse, better, or about the same. Using this item as an index, it was found that approximately 75 per cent of the sample was judged by both raters to be 'about the same' for each of the three assessment points. This provides some empirical support for the suggestion that symptom expression should be relatively stable for the sample as a whole. Table 2.7

31

provides correlations between the three assessments for factor and total scores for the BPRS, KRS, and SANS-AF.

Given the nature of the data and the fact that there was a minimum of three months separating the assessments, the magnitude of the test-retest correlations presented in Table 2.7 are noteworthy with all significant at less than the .05 level and approximately 80 per cent of the coefficients being above .5. Although there are exceptions, correlations are, as would be expected, higher for assessments more closely separated in time. This is especially apparent for the KRS where the mean correlations for assessments one versus two and two versus three (both comparisons separated by three months) are .70 and .60, respectively, while the mean of the coefficients for assessment one versus three (separated by six months, approximately) is .49.

Table 2.7
Test-retest correlations between three assessment points

	Assessment Points		
BPRS	1 vs 2	1 vs 3	2 vs 3
Anxiety-Depression	.66	.84	.71
Anergia	.47	.54	.75
Thought Disturbance	.81	.55	.63
Activation	.71	.65	.68
Hostile-Suspiciousness	.68	.40	.47
Total Score	.77	.63	.57
KRS			
Anxious- Depressed	.76	.38	.43
Poverty of speech	.57	.76	.73
Thought Disorder	.72	.33	.66
Total Score	.74	.48	.57
SANS-AF			
Total Score	.61	.64	.63

The coefficients presented in Table 2.7 should also be interpreted with the understanding that very high correlations (above .9) are not desirable for these sorts of data, i.e., the rating scale may not be sufficiently sensitive to detect change. In view of this and in conjunction with; 1) the fact that 25 per cent of the sample at the time of each assessment was rated by care staff as being either better or worse than usual; and, 2) the knowledge that there was good to very good inter-rater reliability for all of the factor and total scores at all three assessment points, the majority of the test-retest reliabilities are well within an acceptable range.

Having established the scales employed were reliable, correlations were computed between factor scores of each scale and comparable scores across the three rating scales as a means of assessing convergent and discriminant validity (Campbell & Fiske, 1959). Table 2.8 presents these coefficients. The correlation between the total scores of the BPRS and KRS was .87. As can be seen from Table 2.8, correlations between the Anxious-Depressed, Anergia/Poverty, and Thought Disturbance/Disorder factor scores from the BPRS and KRS were .80, .82, and .91, respectively.

These correlations are very high and indicate the scales are measuring similar constructs. However, one other possible interpretation is that the correlations are spuriously high since the ratings scales were completed at the same time, i.e., ratings on one may have influenced the other ratings. As a means of testing this alternative interpretation, correlations were computed between comparable factor scores from the initial assessment point and the first retest. Correlations between BPRS Anxiety-Depression, Thought Disturbance, and Anergia factor and Total scores from the initial assessment and KRS Anxious-Depressed, Thought Disorder, and Poverty factor and Total scores from the first retest were .58, .74, .42, and .64, respectively. The BPRS Anergia factor and the KRS Poverty factor scores from the initial assessment correlated .55 and .59, respectively, with the SANS-AF Total score at the first retest. Although lower than the correlations between equivalent factors from the same assessment point (see Table 2.8), these across assessment points coefficients suggest there is not an insubstantial amount of common or shared variance between scales. Indeed, the correlations between different, but comparable, factor scores from the three scales across assessment points are not too dissimilar to correlations between scores for the same factor across assessment points (see test-retest correlations in Table 2.7).

Table 2.8
Correlations of factor scores within and between the
BPRS, KRS and SANS-AF
Coefficients in bold type significant at less than .005

| | BPRS Factors | | | | KRS Factors | | | SANS-AF |
	Anergia	Thought Disturbance	Hostile Suspicious	Activation	Depressed Anxious	Poverty of speech	Thought Disorder	Total Score
Anxiety- Depression	.01	**.61**	**.58**	.10	**.80**	-.11	**.57**	**-.16**
Anergia		.00	.03	.10	.22	**.82**	-.03	**.96**
Thought Disturbance			**.55**	-.13	**.52**	-.16	**.91**	-.15
Hostile Suspicious				.06	**.50**	-.09	**.58**	-.09
Activation					**.39**	.15	-.10	.03
Depressed Anxious						.10	**.44**	.00
Poverty of speech							-.16	**.86**
Thought Disorder								-.17

The overall pattern of correlations presented in Table 2.8 demonstrates two other important aspects. First, there is good convergence between symptom groups which would be expected to be related. For example, the correlations between the 'neurotic' symptoms of anxiety/depression and hostile/suspicious and the positive symptoms of thought disturbance/disorder are in agreement with the observation that many patients experiencing delusions and hallucinations also "... describe a full range of neurotic syndromes... (and) ... are often depressed, anxious, tense, worried, irritable, distractible, hypochondriacal, and complain of a variety of aches and pains" (Wing, 1978, p. 10). Second, correlations between factor scores which should not be related are low and nonsignificant. The most obvious example being the correlation of .1 between the factors of Anergia and Activation of the BPRS. One other, perhaps somewhat contentious, example is the absence of significant correlations between the positive (Thought Disturbance/Disorder) and negative (Anergia/Poverty/SANS-AF) symptom factors. The finding that all factors are not correlated indicates the ratings are not a function of 'general psychopathology' but are discriminating between symptom clusters.

Table 2.9 presents mean BPRS, KRS, and SANS-AF factor and total scores for the old and new long stay groups for the first administration of each scale. Figures 2.1 and 2.2 display graphically the percent of OLS and NLS subjects rated as exhibiting mild (ratings of 1 or 2), moderate (ratings of 3 or 4), and severe (ratings of 5 or 6) degrees of each symptom for BPRS and KRS. 'Moderate' and 'severe' may be taken to mean 'present to a clinically significant degree' while 'mild' should be interpreted as meaning that, although the symptom in question is present, it is not severe enough to be clinically significant.

Table 2.9
Mean (SD) BPRS, KRS and SANS-AF factor and total scores for
new and old long-stay patients

BPRS	NLS		OLD		Total	
Anxiety-Depression	1.41	(1.33)	0.42	(0.65)	0.70	(1.00)
Anergia	0.92	(1.23)	0.56	(0.68)	0.66	(1.06)
Thought Distance	1.76	(1.63)	0.76	(0.92)	1.05	(1.24)
Activation	0.99	(0.95)	0.75	(1.04)	0.82	(1.01)
Hostile-Suspiciousness	0.78	(0.95)	0.42	(0.69)	0.52	(0.79)
Total Score	19.76	(11.48)	9.04	(8.36)	12.13	(10.48)
KRS						
Anxious-Depressed	1.13	(0.85)	0.48	(0.56)	0.72	(0.75)
Poverty of speech	0.66	(0.85)	0.66	(0.80)	0.66	(0.81)
Thought Disorder	1.39	(1.12)	0.80	(1.02)	0.97	(4.56)
Total Score	8.76	(4.53)	5.20	(4.20)	6.23	(4.56)
SANS-AF						
Total Score	5.26	(6.88)	6.10	(7.88)	5.84	(7.53)

The BPRS factor scores were entered initially into a multivariate one-way analysis of variance (MANOVA), i.e., five factor scores by group (OLS vs NLS). This resulted in a significant overall effect of group, $F(5,53) = 3.84$, $p = .005$. Although using mean factor scores, this analysis is equivalent to analysing the Total Score and as can be seen from Table 2.9, the effect of group was due to the NLS patients having significantly higher overall ratings. To decompose this overall effect, scores for each factor were entered into univariate F-tests (each factor by group). Results revealed significant effects for Anxiety-Depression, $F(1,57) = 14.95$, $p < .001$, and Thought Disturbance, $F(1,57) = 8.81$, $p < .005$. (F-values for Anergia, Activation, and Hostile-Suspiciousness were 1.62, .77, and 2.73, respectively, all p's > .05).

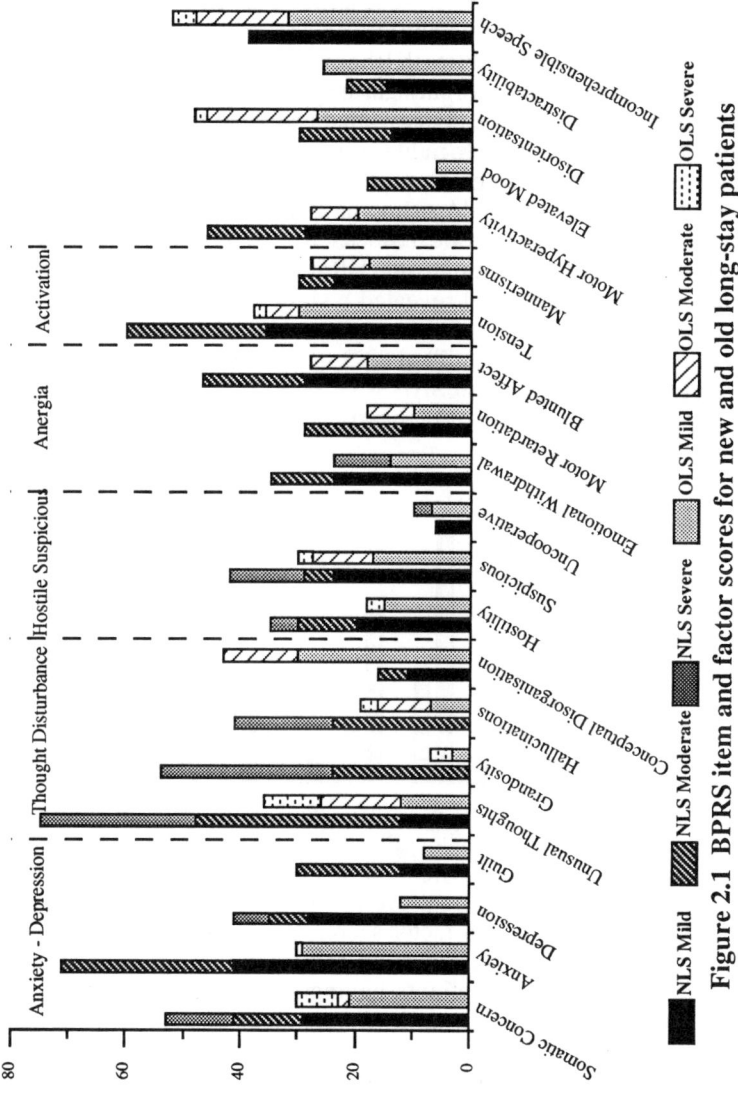

Figure 2.1 BPRS item and factor scores for new and old long-stay patients

To determine which of the individual items were contributing to the differences found for the two factors, Mann-Whitney U tests were performed for each item which contributed to the factor score. For Anxiety-Depression, results were significant for Anxiety, Guilt Feelings, and Depressive Mood with Somatic Concern approaching significance (p = .06). Significant results were found for three (Grandiosity, Hallucinations, and Unusual Thought Content) of the four items of the Thought Disturbance factor with the remaining item (Conceptual Disorganization) approaching significance (p = .06). Analyses of the items Disorientation, Motor Hyperactivity, Elevated Mood, Distractability, and Incomprehensible Speech, which were not included in the five factor scores, revealed a significant effect for Incomprehensible Speech, only.

An initial one-way MANOVA using the three factor scores of the KRS found a significant overall effect of group, F(3,55) = 6.27, p = .001. Results of univariate analyses of the KRS factor scores complimented those found for the BPRS and revealed a significant effect for Anxious-Depressed, F(1,57) = 19.35, p < .001 and the effect for Thought Disorder approaching significance, F(1,57) = 3.89, p = .053. (F-value < 1 for the factor of Poverty).

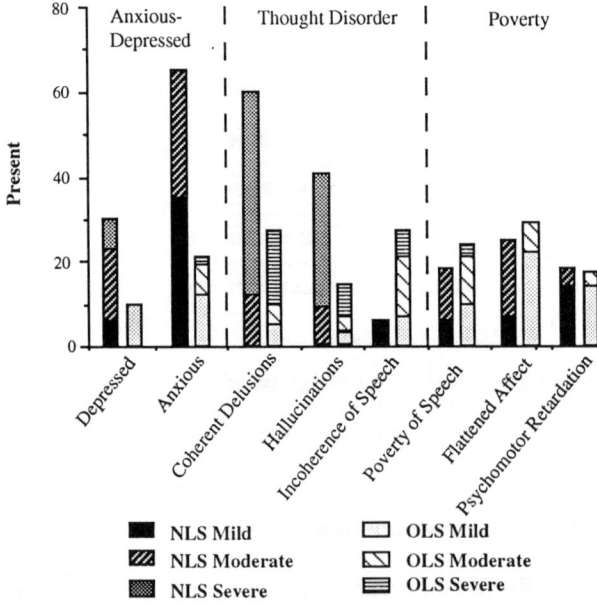

Figure 2.2 KRS item scores for new and old long-stay patients

Using the Mann-Whitney U test, significant differences were found between groups for the items of Depressed and Anxious which comprised the Anxious-Depressed factor. Significant differences between groups were also found for the items of Coherent Delusions and Hallucinations of the Thought Disorder factor. The effect for the remaining item, Incoherence of Speech, contributing to the Thought Disorder factor was not significant.

The total SANS-AF score was not significantly different between groups (F-value < 1). From these results and by reference to Figures 2.1 and 2.2 there appears to be a general trend of a higher proportion of the NLS group reporting some degree of each symptom. In addition, when present, the symptom was rated as being of greater intensity or more severe. This is especially apparent for the affective (anxiety and depression) and positive (hallucinations and delusions) symptoms. This may be due to the differences in ages of these two groups, i.e., a decrease in the number and intensity of symptoms is associated with advancing age (e.g., Bridge, Cannon, & Wyatt, 1978; Lyketsos, Richardson, Aritz, & Lyketsos, 1989). What is somewhat surprising however is the absence of an increase in the number of residual or 'negative' symptoms (e.g. Blunted Affect, Emotional Withdrawal) in the OLS group; these symptoms have been reported to be increase with chronicity (e.g., Ciompi, 1987; Fenton & McGlashan, 1991; Pfohl & Winokur, 1982).

In contrast to the general trend of a higher proportion of NLS patients being rated as exhibiting each symptom, there were more OLS patients who were rated on the BPRS as having some degree of Conceptual Disorganization, Disorientation, and Incomprehensible Speech (see Figure 2.1), and Incoherence of Speech on the KRS (see Figure 2.2). Conceptual Disorganization and Incoherence of Speech were ratings of how confused, disconnected, or disorganized the individual's speech was, while Incomprehensible Speech was rated for the degree to which communication is difficult due to muttering, mumbling, indistinctness, mouthing, whispering, etc'. The finding that these two symptoms, along with that of Disorientation (degree to which the individual was oriented to time, place, and person), were rated as more prevalent and severe in the OLS group may also be due to the age difference between the groups, i.e., more 'organic' type impairments. Interestingly, ratings of clinically significant levels of disorientation were largely due to 'age disorientation'; a discrepancy between subjective and true age (Crow, 1990).

To assess for the stability of ratings over time, each of the factor and total scores from the BPRS and KRS for the three assessment points were entered into a repeated measures ANOVA. After correction to degrees of freedom using the method recommended by Greenhouse and Geisser (1959), no significant effect of assessment occasion was found, i.e., no significant change in symptom ratings over time.

Due to logistic problems, double ratings for the REHAB could not be obtained for twelve patients. Inter-rater reliability estimates were therefore computed from a sample of 52 patients. Degrees of freedom were also reduced by one for items on the REHAB which involved ratings of speech because one patient was mute.

Table 2.10 presents Kappa (K) values for ratings of Deviant Behaviours on the REHAB and intra-class correlation coefficients (ICC) for ratings of General Behaviour items. Intra-class correlation coefficients for the five REHAB factors of Social Activity, Speech Disturbance, Self Care, Community Skills, and Speech Skills were .72, .79, .80, .80, and .58, respectively, and .82 for Total General Behaviour. Although four of the z values (critical z = 1.96 for p < .05) are statistically significant, as can be seen from the K values presented in Table 2.10, only three (Incontinence, Violent, and Shouted at Others) of the seven Deviant Behaviour items of the REHAB demonstrated what would be considered adequate inter-rater reliability.

Table 2.10
ICCs and Kappa values for ratings on the REHAB

	ICC Kappa	z-Value/* F-Value REHAB
Deviant Behaviours		
Incontinence	.85	5.74
Violent	.64	3.23
Hurt Self	–	–
Sexually Offensive	.32	1.49
Absent Without Permission	.07	.31
Shouted at Others	.50	4.92
Laughed to Self	.33	2.99
General Behaviours		
Mixing on Ward	.35	2.07
Mixing off Ward	.70	5.65
Use of Spare Time	.59	3.83
How Active	.57	3.71
How Many Words	.49	2.95
Initiated Conversations	.56	3.52
Sensible Speech	.66	4.82
Clarity of Speech	.74	6.66
Table Manners	.58	3.76
Washed Self	.65	4.78
Dressed Self	.64	4.49
Looked After Things	.71	5.86
Amount of Prompting	.61	4.08
Management of Money	.77	7.77
Use of Public Facilities	.68	5.32
Overall Rating	.62	4.27

*z-Values for Kappa; F-Values for ICCs

Kappa could not be meaningfully calculated for the item Hurt Self due to the low incidence of this behaviour in the sample; only two individuals were rated as having exhibited this behaviour over the last week and in both cases there was disagreement between raters. It is interesting to note that had per cent agreement been used as an index of inter-rater reliability, it would have been reported that raters agreed 96% of the time in ratings of Hurt Self and the inference drawn that ratings of this item were reliable. However, the only valid conclusion that can be drawn is that agreement on its absence is extensive but there is insufficient evidence to suggest ratings of this behaviour are reliable when it does occur.

Although there was good agreement in ratings of Absent Without Permission when it did not occur (80%), raters did not agree on its presence. In fact, there was complete disagreement (hence the K of .07) when at least one of the raters reported its presence. This was not simply due to raters disagreeing on the frequency of occurrence, i.e., once a week or more than once in the past week, since in eight of the ten cases where one rater reported its presence, the other rater reported the behaviour had not occurred in the past week. It is difficult to know why raters do not agree on the presence of this behaviour since the criteria provided by Baker and Hall (1983) are relatively explicit. However, it could be due to interpretation of statements like 'returning an hour or more later than an agreed time' or, the behaviour occurring when one of the raters was on duty while the other was off duty. The latter explanation raises a more general problem with use of the REHAB. This being that, although every attempt was made to choose two members of staff who would be able to observe individuals during the same time window, when working in an active care unit it is not always possible to obtain two key workers who have complete overlap in duty rotas. This is especially problematic when ratings are required for behaviours which occur infrequently.

In addition to divergent time sampling, the poor agreement for ratings of the behaviours Sexually Offensive and Laughed/Talked to Self may be due more to rater differences in interpretation of the criteria for these items. Staff had some difficulty in accepting some of the descriptions of 'sexually offensive' as given by Baker and Hall (1983), e.g., leaving a lavatory door open. Also, although Baker and Hall state that this particular behaviour should be judged 'as if you were a stranger to the ward', staff often build-up tolerances to particular behaviours which would not be acceptable to members of the general community. Another issue which arose when this item was being rated was that the ward/hospital is the patient's 'home'. The point being that behaviours which might be considered sexually offensive in public are not considered to be so in one's own home and given that the hospital or ward is the patient's home then acts such as these should not be considered offensive; patients should not be penalized because of inadequate provisions for privacy. Although ratings on Talked/Laughed to Self are to be done without consideration of the cause or reason, some staff tended to base their ratings on whether or not they thought this particular behaviour was due to underlying pathology; the behaviour was rated as present only when they thought the patient was deluded or hallucinated.

From Table 2.10 it can be seen that, overall, inter-rater reliability for the General Behaviour items of the REHAB is quite good and all are significant at the .01 level or better. The one exception being Mixing on the Ward which, with a ICC of .35, would be interpreted as demonstrating poor agreement between raters. The poor agreement for this item may be due to how the raters interpret 'mixing' and 'gets on well with a good proportion of other patients'. Some staff may take these descriptions to mean active involvement with others whereas some may take these to mean even passive involvement, i.e., simply sitting with others and not creating problems.

Of the instruments used in the present research, the REHAB has been the most extensively evaluated for inter-rater reliability (e.g., Baker, 1986; Carson, Coupar, Gill, & Titman, 1988). In general, the values presented in Table 2.10 are comparable to those published by Baker and Hall (1983) in the REHAB manual with reliability coefficients ranging from .61 to .88 for ratings of Deviant Behaviours and .62 to .92 for General Behaviour items. Unfortunately, the values reported by Baker and Hall are Spearman correlation coefficients and therefore subject to the same criticisms outlined in discussing the psychiatric rating scales (see above). The use of Spearman correlations is especially problematic for Deviant Behaviour items for which there are few scoring categories and where there may be a very high proportion of 'no occurrence'. This has been demonstrated by Baker and Hall (1983) who reported a K value of .27 for the total Deviant Behaviour items reported above, i.e., items which had Spearman correlations ranging from .61 to .88. Unfortunately, they did not report K values for individual items. It would seem however that the values reported in Table 2.10 for the Deviant Behaviour items compare very favourably with Baker and Hall's results. As might be expected, the Spearman correlations reported by Baker and Hall for General Behaviour items are consistently higher than the ICCs listed in Table 2.10. However, the differences are, overall, not very marked; suggesting that, had Baker and Hall used ICCs for their analyses, inter-rater reliability would be equivalent between the original standardization data and the present study.

Table 2.11 presents test-retest correlations for the REHAB factor and Total scores. As can be seen, the correlations between assessment points for each factor are very consistent with all but one being in the .6 to .7 range. Given that these correlations are based on observations for a one week period, separated by a minimum of three months, the results are suggestive of relatively stable patterns of behaviour which can be rated reliably.

Table 2.12 presents correlations between factor, Overall Behaviour, and Total Deviant Behaviour scores. As can be seen from Table 2.12 there are moderate and reasonably consistent significant correlations between the five factor scores of the REHAB.

Table 2.11
REHAB factor scores and total general behaviour score, comparing assessment points

	1 vs 2	1 vs 3	2 vs 3
Social Activity	.76	.78	.62
Speech Disturbance	.47	.68	.68
Speech Skills	.69	.76	.60
Self Care	.69	.71	.63
Community Skills	.71	.68	.65
Total General Behaviour	.72	.79	.62

(All p's <.001)

The very high correlation (r = .81) between Social Activity and Speech Skills is spuriously inflated due to the two items (Amount of Speech and Initiation of Speech) which make-up this factor also contributing to the Social Activity factor.

Table 2.12
Correlations between REHAB scores

	SD	SC	SS	CS	OB	Total Deviant Behaviour
Social Activity	.45	.44	.81	.60	.53	.20
Speech Disturbance (SD)		.52	.47	.31	.52	.47
Self Care (SC)			.49	.46	.60	.48
Speech Skills (SS)				.53	.42	.16
Community Skills (CS)					.49	.26
Overall Behaviour (OB)						.44

As mentioned, the mean of two raters was used for analyses of REHAB items. For individuals for whom only one rating was obtained, this one score was taken to represent a 'mean' score. Degrees of freedom vary in the results reported below because items involving ratings of 'speech', and hence factor scores computed from these, could not be done due to subjects being mute.

Table 2.13
Means (SD) for the five REHAB factors and total scores for the NLS and OLS groups individually and combined, norms taken from Baker and Hall (1983)

	NLS		OLS		Total		Norms	
Social Activity	20.78	(10.86)	26.51	(13.11)	24.88	(12.58)	26.96	(14.63)
Speech Disturbance	3.86	(3.78)	5.73	(4.28)	5.15	(4.18)	5.25	(4.95
Self Care	12.56	(9.78)	18.29	(11.65)	16.78	(11.33)	13.66	(13.10)
Community Skills	5.42	(4.18)	10.55	(5.55)	9.16	(5.64)	9.85	(6.14)
Speech Skills	4.56	(4.73)	6.74	(4.88)	6.12	(4.86)	6.94	(5.17)
Total General Behaviour	47.00	(23.80)	65.90	(29.45)	60.53	(28.85)	60.43	(34.64)
Total Deviant Behaviour	1.72	(1.64)	2.72	(2.27)	2.44	(2.14)	1.42	(1.81)

Table 2.13 presents means and standard deviations for factor and total scores of the REHAB for the the total sample and NLS and OLS groups separately. For comparison, Table 2.13 also shows equivalent scores for a sample of 504 long stay patients used by Baker and Hall (1983) in their standardization of the REHAB. In terms of age and length of present stay, the present sample is similar to that of Baker and Hall's; mean age of the latter was 59 with a range of 19 to 88 years with mean length of present stay ranging from .2 to 64 years and a mean of 18 (see Table 2.3 for equivalent statistics for the present sample). As an aid for interpretation, Figure 2.3 portrays graphically mean scores for items which contributed to each of the factors and, the 'Overall Rating'.

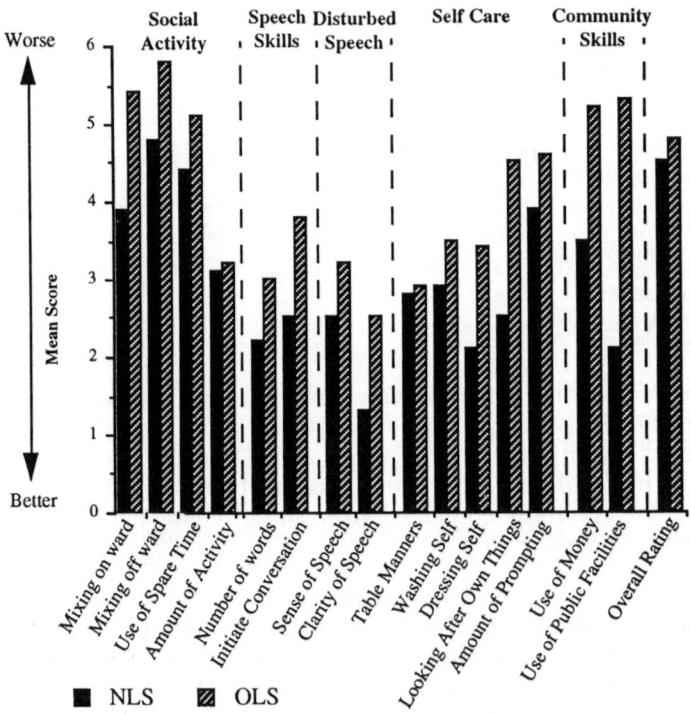

Figure 2.3 REHAB item scores, factors and overall rating for new and old long-stay patients

A 6 (factor scores and Overall Behaviour) X 2 (group) multivariate analysis of variance (MANOVA) of the REHAB data resulted in a significant main effect of group; F(6,54) = 2.87, p = .02. Testing for an overall effect of group in the MANOVA is equivalent to analysing the Total General Behaviour score and as can be seen from Table 2.11 the

OLS patients had a higher mean score. Univariate F-tests of the six REHAB composite scores resulted in one significant difference; that for Community Skills, $F(1,59) = 14.18$, $p < .000$. The effect for Self Care approached significance, $F(1,59) = 3.24$, $p = .077$. The significant effect for Community Skills was due to the OLS group having significantly higher, i.e., worse, scores on this factor. By reference to Figure 2.3, it can be seen that the OLS were rated higher on both items contributing to this factor. However, Mann-Whitney U tests revealed significant differences between groups for the item Use of Public Facilities, only; corrected $z = 3.71$, $p = . 0002$.

A Mann-Whitney U test of the Total Deviant Behaviour score did not reveal a significant difference between the NLS and OLS groups, corrected $z = 1.64$, $p > .05$. The use of a total score for the Deviant Behaviour items is however a rather crude and possibly insensitive means of analysing these data. For example, equal total scores could be the result of very different behaviour patterns, i.e., a score of, say, four for one individual could be due to ratings of two on both Verbal Aggression and Talking to Self while for another the same score could be the result of having been both incontinent and violent more than once in the past week. As a means of investigating the possible confounding effects of using a total score, the per cent of individuals in each group exhibiting at least one occurrence in the past week was calculated for each of the seven deviant behaviours.

Although there appears to be a general trend of a higher proportion of OLS patients being reported as having exhibited each of the deviant behaviours, the only significant difference between the OLS and NLS groups was for Absent Without Permission. This was the one deviant behaviour rated as occurring more frequently in the NLS group. This is not too surprising given that the NLS group was comparatively young and more active and tended to leave the hospital more frequently than OLS patients. In fact, 26 of the OLS patients were living on a 'ward' that was physically isolated with restricted community accessibility.

In contrast to the findings of the psychiatric rating scales, results from ratings on the REHAB indicate a rather homogeneous population. Although there is a general trend for the OLS to be rated as being 'worse' than the NLS, few of these differences reach statistical significance. Further, even for those behaviours where differences are significant, these can be explained by differences in age and environment or location.

Repeated measures ANOVAs on each factor and total score of the REHAB did not reveal any significant differences between the three assessment points carried out in hospital prior to discharge.

Physical health

Table 2.14 presents the number of individuals from the NLS and OLS groups who were rated on the Physical Health Index (PHI) as exhibiting symptoms in the seven systems assessed. The number rated as having a critical disability is also presented. No data were available for seven patients.

It should be noted that five OLS patients and one NLS patient were reported to have symptoms in more than one system and therefore the actual number of individuals exhibiting symptoms of physical disorder in the two groups were 31 (72.1%) and seven (53.8%), respectively.

Table 2.14
Number of NLS and OLS patients exhibiting symptoms in seven physical systems and five critical areas of functioning
In brackets is the number considered to have a 'Disability'

	NLS (N=13)		OLS (N=43)	
System				
Cardiovascular	-		7	
Respiratory	1	(1)	-	
Gastrointestinal Tract	1	(1)	12	(6)
Urogenital	-		4	(2)
Locomotor	-		2	(2)
Central Nervous	4	(4)	9	(8)
Endocrine/Metabolic	2	(1)	3	(1)
Critical Disabilities				
Urinary/faecel incontinence	-		3	
Impaired mobility	-		2	
Blindness	-		1	
Deafness	-		-	
Dyskinesias	-		1	

Although it would appear that there is a larger proportion of OLS who were rated as having a problem in at least one of the physical systems assessed, there is no significant difference ($x2 < 1.0$) between the groups in terms of the proportions considered to have a 'disability'; 15 (34.8%) of the OLS and 6 (46.1%) of the NLS. For the other 16 OLS and one NLS either the disorder was not considered debilitating or there was effective remedial provision. Of the problems rated as a disability, 71% were seen as requiring daily or regular nursing care/supervision.

Seven, or approximately 12% of the total sample assessed, had one of the five critical disabilities. As can be seen from Table 2.14, all seven of these individuals were OLS patients. This is not unexpected given the significant age differences between the groups.

General discussion

The data and analyses presented in this chapter represent the culmination of the selection, piloting, modification, and development of procedures for a comprehensive psychiatric and behavioural assessment to monitor the effects of deinstitutionalisation and community placement on psychiatric patients. This, in conjunction with the other aspects of the study, namely, assessment of Quality of Life (see chapter 6, this volume), treatment environments (see chapter 3, this volume), economic consequences (see chapter 7, this volume), and the longitudinal design employed, makes the present research programme unique. Previous research in this area has been restricted largely to the investigation of only one or two aspects of the possible consequences of resettlement and/or has used, at best, pre-post-discharge designs. Although the findings of the present evaluation may be limited in their generality, it is expected that the comprehensiveness of the assessment procedures will provide valuable insights into the effects and consequences of resettlement.

Reviews of the literature on alternative forms of care to in-patient treatment have called for the experimental investigation of deinstitutionalisation, i.e., the use of control groups and random assignment of subjects to various treatment milieus (e.g., Braun et al., 1981). Although laudable recommendations, there are practical and clinical considerations which, in spite of evaluators' exhortations for the value of true experimental designs, severely restrict their implementation in evaluation research. In the present circumstances, given the political and administrative imperative of rapid resettlement of psychiatric patients and closure of NWH, the development, implementation, and the requisite follow-up period of, at a minimum, one to two years, precluded the experimental evaluation of pilot community programmes. In addition, clinical considerations made untenable the random assignment of patients to the range of community placements to be made available. Indeed, the intended residences and associated levels of support were to be established to cater for the perceived needs of particular groups of patients. With random assignment being impractical, the present evaluation of the resettlement process therefore uses the next best alternative to an experimental design.

In addition to the use of a relatively powerful quasi-experimental design, a notable feature of the evaluation is the attention given to the psychometric properties of the assessment procedures. The majority of the rating scales employed demonstrated at least 'good' inter-rater reliability with coefficients which suggested as good, if not better, agreement between raters than previous published reports. From the results presented it seems that in both absolute and relative terms the assessment instruments have faired very well. This is encouraging and allows for confidence to be placed in the findings. In addition, the policy of continuing to monitor inter-rater reliability at each assessment point and the finding of test-retest reliability estimates in the range not unexpected for the types of measures used, brings added weight to this conclusion.

One further aspect which enhances the current study is the range of subjects included; in terms of age, duration of hospitalisation, psychiatric history, and current symptomatology. The sample includes not only the 'old long-stay' patients but also those who are considered to be the 'new long-stay' or 'young chronic' population. The former being an older group characterised by having spent a large proportion of their lives in psychiatric hospitals and, on the basis of the psychiatric assessments, presently reporting relatively few active or florid psychiatric symptoms, while the latter group is one comprised of relatively young individuals with frequent, relatively brief periods of hospitalisation and who report more positive symptoms.

As suggested previously, the lower incidence of florid symptomatology in the OLS group may be a function of advancing age, i.e., Fewer and less intense symptoms in older patients. However, one other possible explanation is that more OLS patients simply deny or fail to report symptoms that are in fact present. Indeed, the proportion (24%) of the OLS group who admitted to experiencing psychotic symptoms, i.e., hallucinations or delusions, is markedly different from those reported by O'Driscoll et al. (1993) for two large groups of patients similar to the present sample in terms of age and psychiatric history. Depending upon length of stay and hospital, O'Driscoll et al. found 41% to 59% (mean percent of 52) of 'chronic' patients (1 to 20+ years in hospital) scored positively on a 'psychosis' variable. However, in calculating their psychosis score, O'Driscoll et al. included not only self-reported symptoms of hallucinations and delusions but also "whether these either have been noted by staff or are evident from non-verbal behaviour during the interview" (p. 32). Although the present study did not have staff explicitly rate patients for the presence of hallucinations or delusions, one item from the REHAB required staff to indicate whether the patient had been seen to talk or laugh to her/himself. If this item is used as a sign for the presence of hallucinations and/or delusions and the conservative criterion of these behaviours being observed at least twice in the past week adopted, the proportion of individuals in the present OLS sample who would be rated positively for 'psychosis' would rise to 46%; a significant change in proportion (Mcnemar test, p = .002). Although caution must be exercised in inferring the presence of hallucinations or delusions from the observation that an individual talks or laughs to oneself, this value is more in line with those reported by O'Driscoll et al. In fact, if O'Driscoll et al. had used self-reported hallucinations or delusions only as an index of psychosis, the percentage of their sample which would have scored positively on 'psychosis' would have ranged from 32% to 43% with an approximate mean of 37% (see their table 5). Interestingly, the inclusion of the item laughs/talks to self in the calculation of a psychosis score for the NLS group would not increase significantly the proportion who would score positively on this index; 61% versus 67% (Mcnemar test, p > .1). In addition, when staff observational ratings are used as an additional item for ratings for the presence of hallucinations or delusions, there is no longer a significant difference in incidence between the OLS and NLS patients; 46% and 67%, respectively, ($x2(1) < 1$). A similar pattern of results was

46

obtained when data were analysed for only those patients who met the criteria for a DSMIII-R diagnosis of schizophrenia. Whether the lower self-reported incidence of positive symptoms in the OLS group is a function of the natural course of 'schizophrenia', a less stressful environment (i.e., living for a prolonged period in the unchanging inter-personal and physical environment of the long stay ward, little contact with the community, etc.), or simply denial, cannot be known from the present cross-sectional data.

What is interesting is that in spite of the marked differences in psychiatric history and degree of self-reported positive symptomatology, the two groups appear to be rather homogeneous in terms of presence of negative symptoms as rated from behaviour during the psychiatric interview and their rated ability to care for themselves and degree of social activity. Differences that did arise from the behavioural ratings could be accounted for largely by age and environmental factors, i.e., ward environment and location.

The finding of no significant differences between the OLS and NLS groups for ratings of negative symptoms was, as already mentioned, somewhat unexpected. However, it should be noted that not all investigations of the relationship between a deficit syndrome and chronicity have found a higher prevalence of negative symptoms in more chronic samples (e.g., Kay, Fiszbein, Lindenmayer, & Opler, 1986). It would seem that some of the between study variation may be due to methodological differences such as cross-sectional (e.g., Kay et al., 1986) versus longitudinal designs (e.g., Fenton & Mcglashan, 1991) and the ways in which negatives symptoms are operationalized and assessed (Sommers, 1985). Differences in assessment procedure may account for the marked differences in the prevalence of negative symptoms reported by O'Driscoll et al. (1993) as compared to that of the present investigation. Depending upon diagnosis and length of stay, O'Driscoll rated 49% to 75% of the sample as scoring positively on a 'PSE neg' variable. It will be recalled that the percentage of patients in the present study who were rated as exhibiting negative symptoms was considerably lower (see figures 1 and 2). In fact, only 17% of the NLS and 33% of the OLS patients were rated as exhibiting a clinically significant degree of at least one of the negative symptoms from the BPRS (blunted affect, emotional withdrawal) and KRS (flattened affect, poverty of speech). Both blunted affect and flattened affect had to be rated as present to at least a moderate degree for this symptom to be considered present.

In addition to the use of different assessment instruments, there are at least two other possible methodological differences which may account for the discrepancy. First, the presence of negative symptoms in the present study was based only on behavioural observations during the psychiatric interview. O'Driscoll et al. included reports of 'avoidance of social contact' in their 'PSE neg' variable. From results reported by O'Driscoll et al. It cannot be determined the extent to which the inclusion of this item increased the proportion of patients rated for the presence of negative symptoms over that based only on behavioural observations during the interview. As a means of addressing this question, two items from the REHAB ('mixing on the ward' and 'mixing off the ward') were used as indices of 'social contact'. Using a conservative criterion of a score of five or greater for both of these items as indicating reduced social contact and including this as an additional index of a 'negative syndrome' resulted in 28% and 56% of the NLS and OLS patients, or 48% of the total sample, being rated positively for negative symptoms. These values, although still somewhat lower, are more comparable to those reported by O'Driscoll et al. It is noteworthy that when the two REHAB items are included in the computation of a negative symptoms index, a significantly higher proportion of the OLS patients score positively (28% of NLS vs 56% of OLS; $x2(1) = 4.30$, $p < .05$). As with the positive symptoms, restricting this analysis to only patients with a DSMIII-R diagnosis of schizophrenia produced a similar pattern of results. Although the inclusion of 'social contact' items from the REHAB produces results more in line with those reported by O'Driscoll et al., and which would be predicted from at least some of the previous research which has found a higher incidence of negative symptoms in more chronic patients, some caution should be exercised when inferring the presence of a negative syndrome from ratings of the extent to which one interacts with others. As noted by O'Driscoll et al., avoidance of social contact may, in some instances, be due to an active delusional system.

A second possible explanation for the difference between the present study and that of O'Driscoll et al. for incidence of negative symptoms in what appears to be very similar samples is simply a difference in calibration of ratings, i.e., differences between groups of raters in what constitutes a clinically significant degree of a particular sign or symptom. What this means is that although raters within studies may be consistent and demonstrate high inter-rater reliability, there may be differences in expectations and tolerance levels between groups of raters in different studies. In the present investigation, if ratings of 'mild' for negative symptoms observed during the interview are included, 67% and 63% of the NLS and OLS patients, respectively, would score positively. These values are very similar to those reported by O'Driscoll et al.

Overall, it would seem that what appear to be rather marked disparities in incidence of positive and negative symptoms between the present investigation and those of O'Driscoll et al. (1993) are explicable in terms of differences in how the two syndromes were operationalized. Bearing in mind the reservations noted above regarding the use of 'degree of social contact', and inferring the presence of hallucinations and/or delusions from staff observations of 'talking/laughing to oneself', the inclusion of these items as additional indices of negative and positive syndromes, respectively, produces composite scores more comparable to those of

O'Driscoll et al. and, as a result, very similar estimates of the incidence of positive and negative symptoms.

Although not reported in detail here, the suggested divergence of psychiatric and behavioural ratings is supported by the finding of generally low and nonsignificant correlations between factor and total scores of the psychiatric rating scales and the REHAB factor scores. The psychiatric ratings which did tend to correlate with the behavioural ratings were those for negative symptoms, i.e., BPRS Anergia, KRS Poverty, and the SANS-AF. For the total sample, correlations were moderate with the highest mean correlations of the three negative symptom ratings with Social Activity, Speech Skills, and Total General Behaviour being .4, .47, and .33, respectively.

Overall, the results indicate the presence of positive symptoms is unrelated to the perceived level of social activity and extent to which the individual is seen to be able to perform basic activities necessary for independent living. In contrast, there is some indication of a relationship between negative symptoms and degree of behavioural/social disability.

One intriguing and important question which arises from this finding is that of the nature of the relationship. Are the behavioural and social disabilities the effects of institutionalisation (Wing & Brown, 1970)? Or are the negative symptoms due to a disease process with the behavioural disabilities secondary to the lack of motivation and interest associated with the negative syndrome? Although the present data cannot address this issue directly, the finding that the NLS and OLS patients were not significantly different for observed negative symptomatology during the interview and only marginally so for behavioural/social disability suggests that if these deficits are due to the effects of institutionalisation, these must develop at a relatively early stage of hospitalisation, or at least must be carried over from previous periods of hospitalisation.

As a means of exploring further the relationship between negative symptoms, behavioural/social disabilities, and hospitalisation, stepwise multiple regression analyses were conducted. The first used the Anergia factor score from the BPRS as the dependent variable and age, length of present stay, and total years hospitalized as independent variables. Results of the analysis for Anergia indicated that none of the three independent variables entered in the regression analysis were significant predictors of negative symptoms. (A similar result was found in an equivalent analysis of the Poverty factor of the KRS.) In contrast, in a second regression analysis using the Total General Behaviour score of the REHAB as the dependent variable and age, length of present stay, total years hospitalized, Thought Disturbance and Anergia factor scores from the BPRS as independent variables, length of present stay and Anergia were found to account for a significant proportion of the variance (adjusted R2 of .17 or 17%). Although the amount of variance which length of stay and Anergia account for is not overly impressive, 13% and 7%, respectively, the results of this analysis suggest the behavioural and social deficits as rated by the

REHAB are related to the length of time spent in hospital. However, there is also a small but significant and independent contribution of negative symptoms to the explained variance. The results of these exploratory analyses are intriguing but should be treated with circumspection given that only 15 to 20 percent of the total sample exhibited one or more of the negative symptoms during the psychiatric interview at a 'clinically' significant level.

The findings of the psychiatric and behavioural assessments have implications for treatment strategies, support systems required, and future community tenure of the patients included in the resettlement programme. It is clear that many of the OLS and NLS patients have behavioural and social deficits which would restrict their ability to function at a level adequate for independent living. Irrespective of whether the deficits are the result of prolonged hospitalisation or secondary to an underlying pathology, there is an obvious need for, at least initially, continuing support and social and life skills training. Such programmes are necessary if community residences are not to become hospital wards dispersed throughout the community. In fact, there is reason to believe that social and life skills training programmes are beneficial since it has been reported that younger schizophrenics are often responsive to such intervention strategies (Wallace & Liberman, 1985; Anthony & Liberman, 1986). Whether the OLS patients would, given the chronicity of the disabilities, respond in a similar manner is an empirical question but there is reason for optimism.

Although speculative, it would not be unreasonable to suggest that the probability of successful resettlement would be different for the OLS and NLS patients. The reasoning behind this prediction is that the general population is differentially tolerant of the cluster of symptoms which characterise the two groups of patients. In particular, members of the general public are less willing to tolerate someone who is exhibiting positive symptoms and may react critically or even with hostility to an individual who is actively delusional, hallucinating, and behaving in a bizarre manner. Criticism, ridicule, or active rejection may lead to increased levels of stress in the patient as a result of feelings of frustration and/or anger in response to the perceived rejection. Assuming the now commonly accepted diathesis-stress model (e.g., Zubin & Spring, 1977) of major psychiatric disorder is correct, the increased level of stress could very well result in symptom exacerbation and, if sufficiently severe, the need for rehospitalisation. Indeed, this particular scenario could be predicted from the reports of Leff and colleagues (Leff & Vaughn, 1985) on negative expressed emotion. In contrast, the OLS patients who tend not to be overtly psychotic, may not, although perhaps seen as somewhat odd or eccentric, be subjected to the same extent and degree of negative emotions. In addition, the amount of interaction with others may be very different. The OLS patients, being older and probably less active would simply not be exposed to as many potentially negative interpersonal interactions. In addition to the increased probability of the potentially adverse effects of community exposure for the NLS patients, there are the additional problems of non-compliance with treatment and risk for substance abuse and self-injurious behaviours (Minkoff, 1987); problems often associated with younger individuals and a 'revolving-door' pattern of hospitalisation.

The present evaluation by employing a quasi-experimental design which permits many threats to internal validity to be controlled for and the use of assessment procedures which have demonstrable reliability and validity will allow for confidence to be placed in the findings of the resettlement programme. Given the comprehensiveness of the assessment procedures and the range of psychiatric and behavioural disabilities associated with the individuals included, the research will also allow for the investigation of which individuals are best suited for particular community placements/treatment environments. In addition, by employing psychiatric, behavioural, and physical health measures, in conjunction with quality of life and economic assessments, 'outcome' can be evaluated in a number of different ways. Notwithstanding the relatively small sample size, the present group of patients appear to be very similar to the much larger sample of O'Driscoll et al. (1993) in terms of demographic characteristics, psychiatric history, and clinical profiles. In this sense, the individuals involved in the evaluation may very well be 'representative' of the chronic population presently residing in psychiatric institutions. If this is the case, the findings will provide valuable insights and have important implications for programmes of resettlement at other settings.

References

Aldrich, C.K. & Mendkoff, G. (1963), 'Relocation of the aged and disabled: A mortality study', *Journal of the American Geriatric Society*, 11, 185-194.

Alpert, M. (1985), 'The signs and symptoms of schizophrenia', in M. Alpert (ed.), *Controversies in Schizophrenia*. New York: Guilford Press.

Anderson, J., Dayson, D., Wills, W., Gooch, C., Margolius, O., O'Driscoll, C., & Leff, J. (1993), 'The TAPS Project. 13: Clinical and social outcomes of long-stay psychiatric patients after one year in the community', in J. Leff (ed.), 'The TAPS Project: Evaluating Community Placement of Long-Stay Psychiatric Patients', *British Journal of Psychiatry*, 162 (suppl. 19), 45-56.

Andreasen, N.C. (1982), 'Negative symptoms in schizophrenia: Definition and reliability', *Archives of General Psychiatry*, 39, 784-788.

Andreasen, N.C. & Akiskal, H.S. (1983), 'The specificity of Bleulerian and Schneiderian symptoms: A critical reevaluation', *Psychiatric Clinics of North America*, 6, 41-54.

Andreasen, N.C. & Olsen, S. (1982), 'Negative v. positive schizophrenia: Definition and validation'. *Archives of General Psychiatry*, 39, 789-794.

Anthony, A.W., & Liberman, R.P. (1986), 'The practice of psychiatric rehabilitation: historical, conceptual and research base', *Schizophrenia Bulletin*, 12, 542-547.

Avison, W. & Speechley, K. (1987), 'The discharged psychiatric patient: A review of social, social-psychological, and psychiatric correlates of outcome', *American Journal of Psychiatry*, 144, 10-18.

Bachrach, I. (1982), 'Assessment of outcomes in community support systems: Results, problems, limitations', *Schizophrenia Bulletin*, 8, 39-61.

Baker, R. (1986), 'The Development of a Behavioural Assessment System for Psychiatric Inpatients', *Final Research Report to the Grampian Health Board*. Unpublished Manuscript.

Baker, R. & Hall, J. (1983), *Users Manual for Rehabilitation Evaluation of Hall and Baker*. Aberdeen: Vine Publishing Ltd.

Bartko, J. (1976), 'On some reliability coefficients', *Psychological Bulletin*, 83, 762- 765.

Bartko, J. & Carpenter, W. (1976), 'On the methods and theory of reliability', *The Journal of Nervous and Mental Disease*, 163, 307-317.

Bassuk, E.L., & Gerson, S. (1978), 'Deinstitutionalization and mental health services', *Scientific American*, 238, 46-53.

Beck, A., Ward, C., Mendelson, M., Mock, J., & Erbaugh, J. (1962), 'Reliability of psychiatric diagnoses: 2. A study of consistency of clinical judgments and ratings,' *American Journal of Psychiatry*, 119, 351-357.

Bleuler, M. (1974), 'The long-term course of the schizophrenic psychoses', *Psychological Medicine*, 4, 244-254.

Borup, J.H., Gallego, D.T., & Heffernan, P.G. (1980), 'Relocation: Its effect on health, functioning and mortality', *Gerontologist*, 20, 468-479.

Braun, P., Kochansky, G., Shapiro, R., Greenberg, S., Gudeman, J., Johnson, S., & Shore, M. (1981). 'Overview: Deinstitutionalization of psychiatric patients, a critical review of outcome studies', *American Journal of Psychiatry*, 138, 736-749.

Bridge, T.P., Cannon, E., & Wyatt, R.J. (1978), 'Burned-out schizophrenia: Evidence for age effects on schizophrenic symptomatology', *Journal of Gerontology*, 33, 835-839.

Brugha, T.S., Wing, J.K., & Smith, B.L. (1989), 'Physical health of the long-stay mentally ill in the community. Is there unmet need?' *British Journal of Psychiatry*, 155, 777-781.

Campbell, D.T., & Fiske, D.W. (1959), 'Convergent and discriminant validation by the multitrait-multimethod matrix', *Psychological Bulletin*, 56, 81-105.

Carson, J., Coupar, A., Gill, J., & Titman, P. (1988), 'The inter-rater reliability of Hall and Baker's REHAB scale: A cross-validation study', British Journal of Clinical Psychology, 27, 277-278.

Chanfreau, D., Deadman, J.M., George, H., & Taylor, K.E. (1990), 'Transfer of long-stay psychiatric patients: A preliminary report of inter-institutional relocation', *British Journal of Clinical Psychology*, 29, 59-69.

Ciompi, L. (1987), 'Aging and schizophrenic psychosis', *Acta Psychiatrica*, 71, Supplement 319, 93-97.

Cook, T.D., & Campbell, D.T. (1979), *Quasi-Experimentation: Design and Analysis Issues for Field Settings*. London: Houghton Mifflin Co.

Crow, T.J. (1990), 'Meaning of structural changes in the brain in schizophrenia', in, A. Kales, C.N. Stefanis, & J.A. Talbott (eds.), *Recent advances in schizophrenia*. New York: Springer-Verlag.

Dayson, D. (1993), 'The TAPS Project. 12: Crime, vagrancy, death and readmission of the long-term mentally ill during their first year of local reprovision', in J. Leff (ed.), 'The TAPS Project: Evaluating Community Placement of Long-Stay Psychiatric Patients,' *British Journal of Psychiatry*, 162 (suppl. 19), 40-44.

Falloon, I.R.H. (1984), 'Relapse: A reappraisal of assessment of outcome in schizophrenia', *Schizophrenia Bulletin*, 10, 291-299.

Fenton, W.S., & McGlashan, T.H. (1991), 'Natural history of schizophrenia subtypes. II. Positive and negative symptoms and long-term course'. *Archives of General Psychiatry*, 48, 978-986.

Fleiss, J.L. (1981), *Statistical Methods for Rates and Proportions,* 2nd Edition. New York: John Wiley & Sons.

FoxBase+/Mac (1988), *Relational Database Management System.* Perrysburg, Ohio: Fox Software, Inc.

Geller, J.L., Fisher, W.H., Simon, L.J., & Wirth-Cauchon, J.L. (1990), 'Second-generation deinstitutionalization, II: The impact of Brewser v. Dukakis on correlates of community and hospital utilization', *American Journal of Psychiatry,* 147, 988-993.

Goldberg, S., Schooler, N., Hogarty, G., & Roper, M. (1977), 'Prediction of relapse in schizophrenic outpatients treated by drug and sociotherapy', *Archives of General Psychiatry*, 34, 171-184.

Greenhouse, S., & Geisser, S. (1959), 'On methods in the analysis of profile data', *Psychometrika*, 24, 95-112.

Gutmann, G.M. & Herbert, C.P. (1976), 'Mortality rates among relocated extended care patients', *Journal of Gerontology*, 31, 352-357.

Hall, J.N. (1979), 'Assessment procedures used in studies on long-stay patients: A survey of papers published in the British Journal of Psychiatry', *British Journal of Psychiatry*, 135, 330-335.

Hemsley, D.R. (1978), 'Limitations of operant procedures in the modification of schizophrenic functioning: The possible relevance of studies of cognitive disturbance', *Behavior Analysis and Modification*, 2, 165-193.

Honig, A., Pop, P., Tan, E.S., Philipsen, H., & Romme, M.A.J. (1989), 'Physical illness in chronic psychiatric patients from a community psychiatric unit. The implications for daily practice', *British Journal of Psychiatry*, 155, 58-64.

Jasnau, K.F. (1967), 'Individualised versus mass transfer of non-psychotic geriatric patients from mental hospitals to nursing homes, with special reference to the death rate', *Journal of the American Geriatric Society*, 15, 280-284.

Jones, D. (1993), 'The TAPS Project. 11: The selection of patients for reprovision', in J. Leff (ed.), 'The TAPS Project: Evaluating Community Placement of Long-Stay Psychiatric Patients', *British Journal of Psychiatry*, 162 (suppl. 19), 36-39.

Jones, K. (1988), *Experience in Mental Health: Community Care and Social Policy.* London: Sage Publications.

Judd, C.M., Smith, E.R., & Kidder, L.H. (1991), *Research Methods in Social Relations* (6th ed.), Fort Worth: Holt, Rinehart, & Winston, Inc.

Kay, S.R., Fiszbein, A., Lindenmayer, J.P., & Opler, L.A. (1986), 'Positive and negative syndromes in schizophrenia as a function of chronicity,' *Acta Psychiatrica Scandinavica*, 74, 507-518.

Krawiecka, M., Goldberg, D., & Vaughan, M. (1977), 'A standardized psychiatric assessment scale for rating chronic psychotic patients', *Acta Psychiatrica Scandinavica*, 55, 299-308.

Leff, J. (1993), 'Evaluating the transfer of care from psychiatric hospitals to district-based services, in J. Leff (ed.), The TAPS Project: Evaluating Community Placement of Long-Stay Psychiatric Patients', *British Journal of Psychiatry*, 162 (suppl. 19), 6.

Leff, J., & Vaughn, C. (1985), *Expressed Emotion in Families*. New York: Guilford Press.

Leff, J. & Wing, J. 'Trial of maintenance therapy in schizophrenia', *British Medical Journal*, 3, 599-604.

Lowe, C.F., Grant, G., Morell, J.B., Alladin, W.J., & Ellis, N.C. (1988), *Evaluation of the Mental Health Community Service in Clwyd: A Research Proposal*. Unpublished manuscript.

Lukoff, D., Liberman, R.P., & Nuechterlein, K.H. (1986), 'Symptom monitoring in the rehabilitation of schizophrenic patients', *Schizophrenia Bulletin*, 12, 578-602.

Lyketsos, G.C., Richardson, S.C., Aritz, S.K., & Lyketsos, C.G. (1989), 'Prospects of rehabilitation for elderly schizophrenics', *British Journal of Psychiatry*, 155, 451-454.

McGuffin, P., Farmer, A., & Harvey, I. (1991), 'A polydiagnostic application of operational criteria in studies of psychotic illness: Development and reliability of the OPCRIT system.', *Archives of General Psychiatry*, 48, 764-770.

Minkoff, K. (1987), 'Beyond deinstitutionalization: a new ideology for the post-institutional era', *Hospital and Community Psychiatry*, 38, 945-950.

O'Driscoll, C. (1985), *The Physical Health Index*. Unpublished manuscript.

O'Driscoll, C. (1993), 'The TAPS Project. 7: Mental hospital closure - A literature review of outcome studies and evaluative techniques, in J. Leff (ed.), The TAPS Project: Evaluating Community Placement of Long-Stay Psychiatric Patients', *British Journal of Psychiatry*, 162 (suppl. 19), 7-17.

O'Driscoll, C., & Leff, J. (1993), 'The TAPS Project. 8: Design of the research study on the long-stay patients, in J. Leff (ed.), The TAPS Project: Evaluating Community Placement of Long-Stay Psychiatric Patients', *British Journal of Psychiatry*, 162 (suppl. 19), 18-24.

O'Driscoll, C., Wills, W., Leff, J., & Margolius, O. (1993), 'The TAPS Project. 10: The long-stay populations of Friern and Claybury Hospitals, in J. Leff (ed.), The TAPS Project: Evaluating Community Placement of

Long-Stay Psychiatric Patients', *British Journal of Psychiatry,* 162 (suppl. 19), 30-35.

Overall, J. & Gorham, D. (1962), 'The Brief Psychiatric Rating Scale', *Psychological Reports,* 10, 799-812.

Overall, J. & Gorham, D. (1976), 'The Brief Psychiatric Rating Scale in psychopharmacologic research, in W. Guy (ed.),' *ECDEU Assessment Manual for Psychopharmacology.* DHEW Pub. No. (ADM) pp. 158-169. Rockville, MD: National Institute of Mental Health.

Pfolh, B. & Winokur, G. (1982), 'Evolution of symptoms in institutionalised hebephrenic/catatonic schizophrenics', *British Journal of Psychiatry,* 141, 567- 572.

Sommers, A.A. (1985), ''Negative symptoms': Conceptual and methodological problems', *Schizophrenia Bulletin,* 11, 364-379.

Soni, S., Soni, S.D., & Freeman, H.L. (1978), 'Group homes for psychiatric patients. An evaluation of six years' experience in the domestic resettlement of chronic psychiatric patients', *International Journal of Mental Health,* 6, 66-79.

SPSS Inc. (1988), *SPSS-X User's Guide.* Chicago: SPSS Inc.

Thornicroft, G., & Bebbington, P. (1989), 'Deistitutionalisation-from hospital closure to service development', *British Journal of Psychiatry,* 155, 739-753.

Vaughn, C. & Leff, J. (1976), 'The influence of family and social factors on the course of psychiatric illness: A comparison of schizophrenic and depressed neurotic patients', *British Journal of Psychiatry,* 129, 125-137.

Wallace, C.J., & Liberman, R.P. (1985), 'Social skills training for patients with schizophrenia: a controlled clinical trial', *Psychiatry Research,* 15, 239-243.

Weller, M.P. (1989), 'Mental illness - who cares?' *Nature,* 339, 249-252.

Wing, J. (1968), 'Social treatments of mental illness', in M. Shepherd & D. Davies (eds.), *Studies of Psychiatry.* London: Oxford University Press.

Wing, J.K. (1971), 'How many psychiatric beds?' *Psychological Medicine,* 1, 188-190.

Wing, J. (1975), 'Impairments in schizophrenia: A rational basis for social treatment,' in R.D. Wirt, G. Winokur, & M. Roff (eds.), *Life History Research in Psychopathology.* Minneapolis, MN: University of Minnesota Press.

Wing, J.K. (1978), 'Clinical concepts of schizophrenia', in J.K. Wing (ed.), *Schizophrenia: Towards a New Synthesis.* London: Academic Press.

Wing, J.K. (1983), 'Use and misuse of the PSE', *British Journal of Psychiatry,* 143, 111-117.

Wing, J.K., & Brown, J. (1970), *Institutionalism and Schizophrenia.* London: Cambridge University Press.

Wing, J.K., Cooper, J., & Sartorius, N. (1974), 'The Description and Classification of Psychiatric Symptoms', *An Instruction Manual for the PSE and CATEGO system*. London: Cambridge University Press.

Wykes, T. (1982), 'A hostel-ward for 'new' long-stay patients: An evaluative study of a 'ward in a house',' in J.K. Wing (ed.), 'Long-Term Community Care: Experience in a London Borough', *Psychological Medicine Monograph Supplement 2*. Cambridge: Cambridge University Press.

Zubin, J., & Spring, B. (1977), 'Vulnerability - a new view of schizophrenia', *Journal of Abnormal Psychology*, 86, 103-126.

3 The care process: Care environments, care management and staff attitudes

Charles Crosby, Michael F. Carter and Margaret M. Barry

Summary

In this chapter the process of care is examined in hospital and two community residential schemes. Three main themes are identified which contribute to the outcomes of care - care environment, care management and staff attitudes. Each of these has a part to play in determining the levels of social and behavioural functioning which individuals achieve. Care Practices are shown to be less restrictive in the community schemes than in hospital. In one ward housing old long-stay patients levels of social interaction were found to be particularly low. Planning in both hospital and community emphasises the importance of implementing individual action plans (IAPs) as a means of making care management systematic. Such plans are particularly important in the preparation of individuals for transfer from hospital to the community. However, plans are not always fully implemented, especially in wards for old long-stay patients, and the follow through of hospital planning to the community may be only partial. Hospital staff attitudes to community care reveal some hopes that there might be improvements for patients, coupled with doubts about the adequacy of community care and fears for job security in the future. Twelve months after the transfer to the new care settings community staff are positive about the benefits for clients of the new forms of care. However, a strong need for training was expressed by unqualified community staff, chiefly in order to gain an understanding of problem behaviours in clients and to develop care management skills.

Care environments are shown to be important in expressing the objectives of the care philosophies to be practiced in them. Small scale, domestic environments, which afford privacy and accessibility, provide an opportunity framework for individual development which was lacking in hospital.

Introduction

The Victorian asylums were the physical expression of the philosophy and aims of the system of psychiatric care which gave rise to them (Murphy, 1991). In the second half of the twentieth century in Britain movements arose which drove towards a revision of psychiatric care management. These rendered both the previous physical institutional expressions of care and traditional care practices inappropriate to achieving optimum outcomes for chronic psychiatric patients. Elements which have led to this changed perspective include scientific innovation in medication, (Jones, 1988); societal reactionism (Lemert, 1951, Becker, 1963) which focuses upon the interaction between the deviant and those who apply such labels; anti-institutionalism (Goffman, 1968, Barton, 1959); and economic necessity (Scull, 1979, 1984). The North Wales study has focused upon one experiment in fulfilling these imperatives, in which the concepts of normalisation are partially realised through relocation of chronic, long-stay patients into accommodation which is domestic rather than institutional and care management is modelled on developments which have followed the 1990 National Health Service and Community Care Act. In these circumstances care management, staff attitudes and the qualities of the residential environment form a loosely structured model of care which is directed toward improving outcomes for clients. Care management has become the vehicle through which an integrated, seamless service will be delivered in these new settings, rather than the unitary integration of the hospital provider.

The concepts of 'care management' and 'case management' are currently the subject of much discussion, and the focus of important research initiatives (for example, Ford et al., 1993). It is by no means clear that agreed definitions of the components of each term exist. Broadly, case management is concerned with the coordination of all aspects of the care process, from client identification and engagement through the preparation of individual action plans and the coordination of service delivery to monitoring and evaluation. The case manager is primarily concerned with the identification of need, the organisation of a package of care and monitoring outcomes and development rather than being involved in direct care provision. The introduction of case management, in parallel with the move from hospital to community based services in Britain, has been a response to the perceived danger of the fragmentation of community mental health services and the possibility of clients 'falling through the net' of care. Models of case management and the extent of its introduction vary widely in England and Wales. The development of models which have wide acceptance is considered to be a necessary step in the provision of coherent community mental health services (Ryan, et al., 1991).

Evaluation aims and methods

Issues concerning care practices, staff attitudes and care environments, have been investigated as part of the North Wales Study of deinstitutionalisation. The aim of this chapter is to describe the factors in each of these areas which contribute to the organisation of care and determine its outcomes for residents in the hospital and in the community. Each of the areas has been identified by planners, managers and care workers, as well as the research team, as being an area of change which will significantly alter the delivery of psychiatric services in North Wales (Clwyd Health Authority, 1991).

The following research instruments were used to investigate care environments, care practices and staff attitudes:-

Care environments

- Architectural Checklist (Robinson et al., 1984)
  The instrument provides a classification on a dichotomous instrument which determines whether environmental features under consideration are primarily institutional or domestic in character.

Care practices

- Hospital and Hospices Practices Profile (Wykes, 1982)
  The instrument provides a scale which measures the degree of restrictiveness in care practices.

- Behavioural Observation Instrument (Alevizos et al., 1978).
  This provides a time sampling procedure for recording the behaviour of persons which can be used to assess the effect of care practices on groups of psychiatric patients.

- Needs Assessment Schedule for Care Staff developed by the research project team. The instrument provides a staff assessment of client needs and a measure of the extent to which these are met. It is based on work by the Personal Social Services Research Unit (1986).

Staff attitudes

- Staff Attitudes and Management Practices Schedule based on work by Garety and Morris (1984). This instrument provides data on staff and management attitudes to care management.

The care settings

Hospital

The North Wales Hospital is a large victorian institution set in extensive grounds approximately one mile outside a small market town. Psychiatric care for both Gwynedd and Clwyd has until recently been focused on the hospital. From a maximum of 1,409 beds in 1964, numbers have now dropped to below 300 patients for the first time in the history of the hospital. Closure has been targeted for 1995, with the reprovision of services through community mental health teams and acute general hospital facilities. The environment of the hospital is largely institutional, with long bare corridors and dormitory wards which afford little privacy being a predominant feature. Overall care management objectives were defined as being to rehabilitate people who have lost everyday living skills, who have to re-establish and reinstate themselves. Staffing levels and qualifications were higher in the rehabilitation wards which mainly accommodate 'new long-stay' patients than the long-stay wards which provide for 'old long-stay' patients who have lived in the hospital for many years. The staff to patient ratio averaged 0.53:1 on old long-stay wards and 0.95:1 on rehabilitation wards.

Community

Community Care Scheme 1 is a registered care scheme run by MIND, providing twenty-four hour support to patients resettled from three of the four hospital wards studied. The scheme provides residential care for ten people in six flats. Each flat has its own kitchen, bathroom, living area, and individual bedrooms. The physical environment is predominantly domestic, but there are some institutional features, such as a communal lounge and staff office accommodation. The average age of the clients resettled here was 48 years and their average length of hospitalisation prior to discharge was approximately 11.5 years. The care staff consists of project workers, one deputy manager and a manager. The scheme opened in November, 1990 and provides community-based residential care which stresses independence and self-development of residents. A key worker system operates. Staff meetings are held monthly for the purpose of providing a focus for inter-staff communication. Staff training is considered a high priority and all staff are encouraged to develop their careers. Most direct care staff were not professionally qualified at the start of the scheme. The staff to client ratio is 1:1.

Community Care Scheme II provides twenty-four hour supported living to fifteen adults, all being former long-stay psychiatric patients resident in the most isolated of the four hospital wards surveyed. The average age of those resident in the scheme was 66 years, and the average length of continuous hospitalisation prior to discharge had been 26 years. The scheme is made up of five houses. Each house provides furnished residential accommodation and has three or four bedrooms. The physical environments are completely domestic. Clwyd Community Care NHS Trust is responsible for provision of twenty-six community support workers, a project manager and one deputy project manager, whose work is divided between management of the scheme and community psychiatric nursing. Care workers in each house form a key worker group. Staff support and training is provided by the managers. The majority of direct care staff are not professionally qualified. The staff to client ratio is 1.6:1.

Care environments

Mental health care has tended to be concerned with practical questions concerning the provision of adequate levels of support. For psychiatric hospital patients the emphasis was on a custodial role, to remove the risks that are part of everyday life in the community and to replace the impaired capacities for self-help with functional care. The large Victorian institutions for the care of psychiatric patients expressed these concerns in characteristic physical forms, which had implications for the nature of the care regime to take place in those forms and which, in turn, impinged on and created an important part of the quality of life for those residents in such institutional settings. An important part of the move from large institutional environments to the provision of care in a variety of new locations is to establish the foundations of care in less institutional and more homely contexts. There has been considerable support for the belief that everyone prefers to 'live in an ordinary house rather than in institutions, because institutions lack the capacity to be a home' (Means and Smith, 1994). Gurney and Means (1993) have suggested that there is debate within urban sociology concerning the significance of home. Part of this discussion has focussed around home ownership and the idea of stratification of the meaning of home for different social groups, relating to the type of tenure, whether owner-occupied council rented or privately rented. The meaning of 'home' for individuals and specific groups in society is by no means clear. Some of the complexities of these issues are discussed by Sixsmith (1986) and Copeland, et al., (1988). At an individual level, home can have many different meanings, and can be valued in different ways, depending on the purposes and motivations of the person.

Evaluating the care environment

The care environments of the four hospital wards and the two community care schemes in this study have been investigated using a checklist of socially significant architectural features, developed by Robinson et al

(1984). The value of this checklist is that it was designed specifically for evaluating the institutional character of residential settings, which are described by dichotomously juxtaposing the physical characteristics of a typical domestic environment against those of a traditional institution. The study was developed to understand the environmental implications of the normalisation principle. While the concept of the normalisation has been a primary factor in the movement toward deinstitutionalisation of psychiatric populations, there had been no systematically developed architectural definition of the term prior to this study.

The study by Robinson et al. provides a comprehensive checklist of the features of residential care environments. The principal of polarity has been followed, and each item on the checklist may be designated as exhibiting principally institutional or principally home-like features. The schema complements the concern of the present study with institutionalisation and the contrast of less institutional environments. The architectural checklist was therefore used to derive a set of socially significant characteristics about care environments which matched the areas of social concern to the research, namely: privacy, independence, the symbolic environment, personalisation and the social environment. For example, items used to assess privacy include individual bedrooms, separation of public areas from the individual's domain, whether toilets are non-communal, the provision of non-communal outdoor space. The presence of each of these features is indicative of a privacy which is domestic, while its absence suggests an institutional environment. The relevant observations on the architectural checklist were completed by a research worker. The ratings on this schedule were whether the characteristics were principally homely, or institutional in accordance with the check list definitions. Where the characteristics contributing to each item were principally homely a score of one is allocated. Where the characteristics are principally institutional the score is zero.

Privacy. The issue of privacy is seen as central by Willcocks, et al. (1987) in a study of residential life in local authority old peoples homes. Booth (1985) notes a number of reasons for the importance of privacy; it can shield the individual who might be vulnerable to the actions and power of others; it offers a space for self-expression and choice, which might be restricted by the constraints of communal living; a private space is needed, because people who are forced to live in public 'may only be able to find the privacy they need by turning in upon themselves'. Although privacy is recognised as a basic human need, there is often a neglect of it, both in the physical characteristics of institutional care and in care practices themselves.

While Clough (1981) had suggested that residential care should provide a 'living base' for residents that is broadly the equivalent of ordinary housing, Higgins (1989) has emphasised the considerable differences between the two. Institutional life lacks privacy and intimacy, while imposing limitations on choice and personal freedom. It is owned by other agencies and residents tend to lack security of tenure. Many informal, daily events and activities take place in the intimacy of the home, such as relaxing, reading a paper or chatting to friends. Institutions generally deprive individuals of the routine of domestic tasks, such as cleaning, cooking and washing up, which may provide a framework for life.

The hospital ward environments afforded a lower degree of privacy (29% of the maximum possible) compared to the two community care schemes (64%). The hospital environment benefited from there being secluded areas and countryside around the building but internally the arrangement of dormitory ward accommodation provided negligible privacy for individuals. In the community schemes the majority of residents had their own bedroom (75%) or shared with one other person (25%) and the use of a living room where they could take visitors.

Independence. the maintenance and restoration of independence is an important theme in mental health care. Attention has been given to the apparent loss of independence associated with institutional accommodation, while ordinary housing is seen to afford independence. At an individual level, the notion of independence may be personally defined and independence and dependence need not be construed as opposites. As Munnichs (1976) points out, for an older person:

> … dependency is only perceptible when changes in his existence which concern himself present themselves or are introduced: relocation, admission to hospital.

This emphasis on the subjective and emotional quality of 'self-integrity' seems to be the key to understanding the human experience of 'independence'. As Fisk (1987) puts it:

> it describes a state of determination whereby the individual, with or without assistance and regardless of disability, is able to dictate the path that his or her life should take. It is a state that is determined both by personality and the individual's social and physical environment.

It is these qualities of self-determination that seem to be absent in institutional settings. This observation is made by Willcocks et al., who develop a critique of residential care based on a comparison with 'domestic' home. They suggest that a key difference lies in the role of domestic home as a 'personal power base and a source of self-identity'. They argue that these qualities can sustain independence. In institutions there seems to be a mutual agreement between carers and residents that the locus of responsibility is with the former. The structure of communal living also tends to inhibit individuality and responsibility through the block treatment of residents. Finally, Willcocks et al., point to the relative absence in institutions of the risk and uncertainty that characterise life within the community. Again, the contract between the carer and the cared- for is based on the compromise of the personal independence that characterises life in the domestic home.

Independence in terms of the care environment is conceived as being the extent to which the building facilitates individual activities, such as access to local facilities (shops, cafés, banks, post office), access to recreational space outside the building, and a usable domestic kitchen. In the hospital access to facilities was restricted by the distance of the building from the town centre and lack of public transport. Access to recreational spaces outside was made more difficult by long corridors and flights of stairs to be negotiated and food was supplied from a large central kitchen. The overall score was 31% of the possible score for a physical environment which promoted independence. Such restrictions were largely absent in the community schemes, with easily accessible shopping facilities, direct access to gardens and modern domestic kitchens available for the residents' use. The total score in these settings was 89%.

The Symbolic Environment. The physical environment of the dwelling may have symbolic attributes as well as purely functional ones. Harrison and Means (1990) analysed the significance of the home for a group of elderly owner-occupiers and found that personal attachment, familiarity and the association of the place with family relations and life events were important to residents. The meanings associated with an environment may be subtle and complex and even the most mundane object may acquire significance.

Robinson et al, (1984) examined the symbolic qualities of residential settings. They argue that many of the cues for behaviour come from the physical environment, and are critical of some of the typical features of institutional accommodation:

> Whereas in institutions, living rooms are generally very large in scale with furniture at the perimeter, in ordinary housing a living room will be small with chairs variously placed, some at right angles for conversation, others isolated near a lamp for reading.

This example has a specific behavioural focus, but one should consider how the features of the environment contribute to behaviour in general. A building that is of primarily institutional character continually reinforces an institutional 'consciousness' and behaviour on the part of carers and residents. Institutional surroundings may provide cues for particular forms of behaviour by staff. For example, many architectural features of institutions have been designed for convenience, such as bathrooms, large kitchens and staff offices. Institutional design may prompt institutional behaviour. Conversely, Robinson et al. argue that a home like setting encourages staff to treat residents in a more normal fashion, because it tends to elicit from both behaviours suitable to home which they have learned and have had reinforced previously in many similar environments.

The character of large dormitory wards, sparsely furnished, with little personalisation or private space, is both symptomatic and creative of much of the depersonalisation which has been evident in large psychiatric hospitals in the past and which still persists at present. It is important to minimise the institutional character of residential care settings. This involves attention to the external and internal structure and appearance of the buildings and the artefacts within it. The movement of patients from large institutional settings into smaller, more homely environments is a part of this process and a recognition of residents as individuals.

The symbolic environment is characterised by features which indicate an institutional environment, such as staff offices, information desks and business premises, while a domestic environment has an absence of these and instead has homely furnishings, ornamental features, and carpeted floors. The hospital environment predominantly symbolised institutional characteristics and scored 25% of the possible score for domestic features. The community schemes were designed to provide domestic environments for residents and achieved a score of 85%.

Personalisation. One aspect of the quality of the environment that has been a central issue is the 'home as a symbol of self' (Rapoport, 1969: Becker, 1973; Cooper, 1972, 1974; Pratt. 1982). This concept developed from an interactionist perspective, which suggested that the place in which a person lives tells something about the person. From this standpoint, the house becomes symbolic of the dweller, not only in the sense of showing others that the house is occupied by someone in particular (Duncan and Duncan, 1976a, 1976b), but also in the sense of reinforcing the occupant's self-conception (Becker 1973: Appleyard, 1979; Rapoport, 1982). The question of how the home reflects or reinforces identity is difficult. People seem to need external assurance of their own identity (Erikson, 1968) and the material manifestation of the house can act in this way. Through personalisation, the home becomes an expression of how the person sees himself and how he would like himself to be seen (Goffman, 1959). Thus, the home may be a necessary component of identity and a sense of self. Interest in this general area has focused on people in institutional settings. Communal living by definition limits the expression of self through the environment. To an extent, a move to an institution can be seen as a surrender of personal self to a self that is socially defined. Because of this, many commentators have emphasised the need for personalisation within residential care in order to promote more 'homelike' settings. In many cases, furniture and personal possessions are displayed prominently, even in cramped circumstances. Whatever the approach adopted by the individual, institutions should offer scope for personalisation, and hence the expression of self.

Personalisation of the residential accommodation in hospital was extremely low. Individuals had few possessions of their own and little opportunity to give personal character to places where they had lived for many years. These environments achieved only 10% of the possible score for personalisation. In contrast, the community settings provided much greater opportunity for personalisation of bedroom and lounge areas and residents were encouraged by staff in this activity. The resultant score of 79% indicates that, given the opportunity and encouragement, residents could re-gain the taste for individualisation of place of residence which is so characteristic of normal domestic environments.

The social environment - Community integration. Many of the issues discussed so far, such as privacy, emphasise the dwelling environment as the domain of the individual, in particular the expression of individual identity through personalisation. Yet it is obvious that most homes are also social units. There are perhaps a number of levels to this social dimension. Firstly, there is the social domain of the house itself. In western cultures, the home as a social unit refers to the nuclear family, and the family unit has its physical equivalent in the dwelling unit (whether this is a house or a flat). Harrison and Means (1990) found the family, in a personal, affective sense, to be a primary dimension of home experience. Participants emphasised the importance of relationships, love and togetherness, a sense of belonging, warmth and security, mutual respect and a feeling of being cared for, as the central meaning of home.

The social dimension of the dwelling environment is also significant at the neighbourhood or community level. Hayward points to the wider social context of the residence which is not only a matter of close personal relationships, but also the social ties and interactions with family members, neighbours and acquaintances. The significance of these interactions lies in their relative permanence and continuity, leading to a sense of familiarity and 'at homeness' within the locale.

Criticism of institutional care has supported the increasing emphasis on domiciliary care (Townsend, 1962; Meacher, 1969; DHSS, 1981). Clough (1981), however, is critical of some of the unqualified assumptions that lie behind the attitude that living in the community is preferable for all people at all times. Models of domiciliary care tend to be idealised, in contrast to the picture of inadequate institutional care. Of more relevance to the present discussion is his comment that the relocation of long-stay residents in less institutional environments needs to be critically examined. It cannot be assumed that home-like environments will always mean the best quality of life for the individual concerned.

In this study the social environment is concerned with the extent to which the location and characteristics of the dwelling are integrated with a residential community. This refers to location in residential areas and the scale and style of the building being compatible with those around it, for example, a detached or semi-detached house in a residential area. The hospital buildings were massive and isolated while the community schemes were well integrated in mainly residential area. Scores on the environmental checklist are respectively 5% and 94%.

Summary

The quality of the environment in the hospital wards was generally poor. Two wards housed 'old long-stay' patients and these had the poorer environments in terms of access to facilities, such as shops and cafés. degree of privacy for residents (dormitory sleeping arrangements), and the maintenance of cleaning, decorating, and repairs. Two rehabilitation wards were better and, in one case, offered better accommodation, including single bedrooms. Generally, the wards achieved only 20% of the potential score for domesticity on the environmental checklist and were highly institutional environments. In contrast two community care scheme which were established to accommodate patients being resettled from hospital were predominately domestic environments, achieving 82% of potential score for domesticity on the environmental checklist. The significance of the change in care management and care environment for clients is clearly illustrated in the comments of one community resident:

> It's a house; I can go in the kitchen for food, I can sit in the lounge, I can go upstairs to my own bedroom. I had none of that in hospital. I have more freedom. I'm supported but I can organise myself here. It's home.

Planning resettlement

In the present study, resettlement of the research cohort from hospital has proceeded in stages. The research cohort was formed in 1989 by the selection of two 'old long-stay' wards and two 'new long-stay' wards, for inclusion in the study. The selection of entire wards meant that it was possible to analyse the care practices in the hospital regimes and compare these with new community settings. Two years after commencement of research, 34 subjects from the cohort of 65 had been resettled and had spent twelve months in the community. Thirty one subjects had remained in hospital. The majority of those resettled (24 subjects - some 70% of the resettlement group) had been relocated to Community Care Scheme I and Community Care Scheme II. Resettlement to other care settings included private care homes for people with mental health problems (4), Social Services homes (2), family living (2) and independent living (2).

The development and implementation of IAPs is the basis of individual care management and ensuring the quality of that care in both hospital and community. In hospital IAPs are developed by multidisciplinary teams and it is rare for clients to participate directly in this process. Examples of the activities which form part of IAPs in hospital include cooking, laundry, shopping and budgeting.

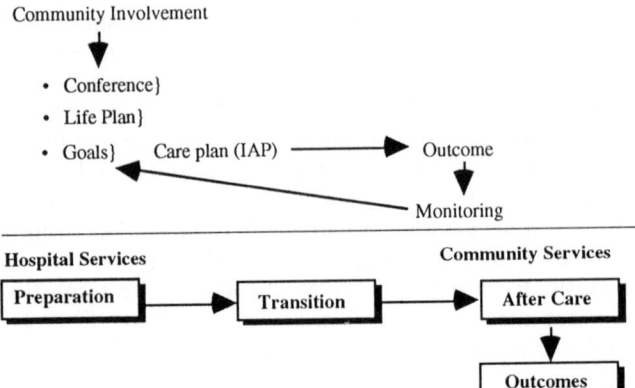

Needs Assessment
- Client Biography
- Client Involvement
- Relatives' Involvement
- Community Involvement

- Conference}
- Life Plan}
- Goals} Care plan (IAP) ⟶ Outcome

Monitoring

Hospital Services   **Community Services**

Preparation ⟶ Transition ⟶ After Care

Outcomes

Figure 3.1
Hospital resettlement planning:The preparation of individual action plans

Leisure activities include adult education, horse riding, swimming, regular trips out and use of the community such as pubs and shops when possible. However, it is notable that while this positive involvement in activities embraces all clients in rehabilitation wards, in one of the old long-stay wards only 4 out of 11 residents actually took part in positive training programmes, while in the other old long-stay ward, it was difficult to identify such plans being put into practice on a coherent basis, except when individual workers were preparing an individual resident for resettlement. In hospital very little decision-making involved clients. Staff reported that no patients were involved in deciding about their programmes of care, although 'contracts' were made with patients to try to establish behavioural standards. The formal process of developing IAPs in hospital is shown in Figure 3.1.

In fact, decisions in the hospital were made by a combination of nursing staff at ward level and senior nursing staff at management level. There was very little decision making between staff and patients with respect to any of the areas questioned. As the process of resettlement of patients developed, there was a tendency for staff on the two old long-stay wards to feel that they were acting merely in a caretaking capacity. A large majority of hospital nursing staff felt that they had not been given training to undertake rehabilitation work and staff became increasingly dissatisfied with the insecurity and lack of opportunity for career advancement. In these circumstances the formal models of resettlement planning and implementation were not closely adhered to.

In addition the process of selection for resettlement was less clearly defined in the two 'old long-stay' wards, particularly in one ward in which care management and the use of IAPs was least developed. In this situation, selection for resettlement and preparation appeared to be more at the discretion of individual nursing staff, who had elected to support the objectives of resettlement and hospital closure and had chosen to work as resettlement nurses. These placements mainly resulted in finding individual places in private homes or social services homes (shown in Figure 3.2). The conclusion of this process of individual placement was that fifteen residents remained, who were all allocated to Community Care Scheme II when the ward was due for closure. In contrast Community Care Scheme I drew clients from the three other wards, but mainly focused on individual selection from the two rehabilitation wards. The result of these selection procedures was that Scheme II was designed to accommodate the residual population of old long-stay patients, while Scheme I acquired mainly new long-stay residents. The planning of community placements is shown in Figure 3.3.

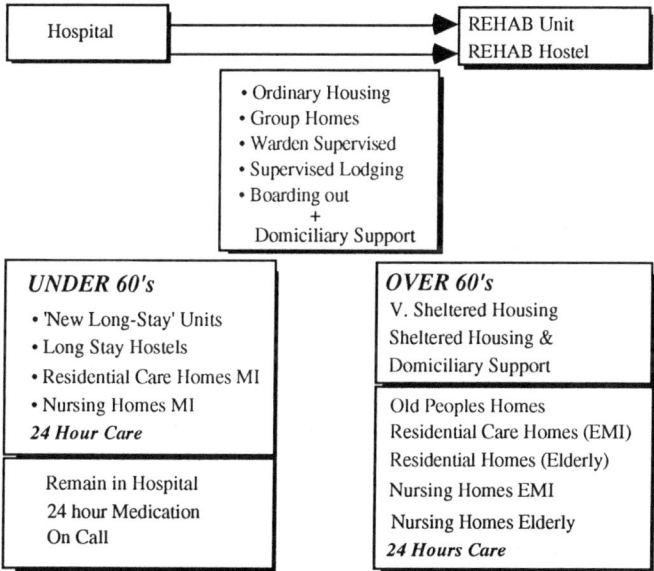

Figure 3.2
Hospital grouping of clients and initial identification of relocation options

71

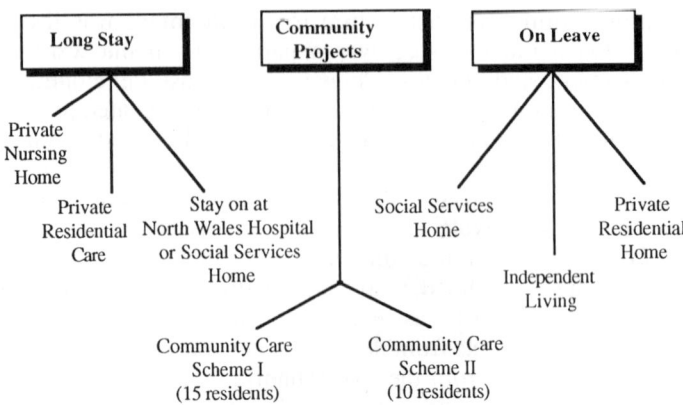

Figure 3.3
Provisional planning of community placements

Hospital and community care practices

The Hospital-Hospices Practices Profile (HHPP) provides a means of assessing the extent to which care management practices allow freedom of choice to the individual or restrict choice by imposing an institutional regime. Following other researchers this study has taken the total score in this scale as an indication of how restrictive the care regime is (Wykes, 1982). The higher the score the more restrictive the care regime.

A schedule of care practices using the HHPP items was completed by a member of the research team with the ward charge nurse on each of the four wards included in the study. The same procedure was followed with the managers of the two community schemes under scrutiny. It should be noted that the HHPP items referred to the ordinary daily practices of the ward or residence and not to special or unusual situations. A rating of zero means that the practice is not normally adopted and a rating of one means that it is. This follows the scoring method adopted by Wing (1982) in comparing residential and day care units.

In Community Care Scheme 1 only 6% of practices were restrictive. (Fig 3.4) The corresponding figure in Community Care Scheme II is 20%, while Hospital Rehabilitation wards had a score of 26% and the 'old long-stay' wards 40%. With a score of 6%, Community Care Scheme I is highly orientated to resident freedom and independence. This is a lower score for restrictive practices than that founded by Richardson (1977) in the most client orientated centre in study of psychiatric day centres for chronic patients. It indicates the strong commitment of management in the scheme to independence for clients. It is important to note that although care management in Community Care Scheme I is less restrictive than that of Community Care Scheme II, residents of both schemes have experienced a

72

substantial reduction in restrictive practices in the move from hospital to community. On the scale used, care management in the community is some 20% less restrictive for residents in both community care schemes than was hospital care management, Scheme II accommodating only those who had previously been resident in an 'old long-stay' ward.

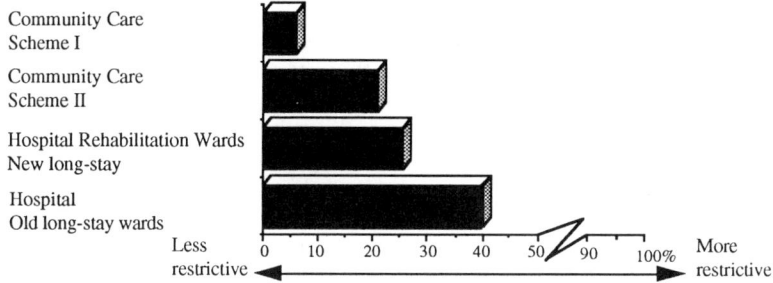

Figure 3.4
Hospital and Community Care Schemes. Hospital-Hospices Practices Profile

Levels of patient engagement

As part of the research programme it was decided to undertake an observational study of patient engagement in what appeared to be the more deprived of the two old long-stay wards. Following an inspection of several possible instruments, an adaptation of the Behavioural Observation Instrument (BOI) of Alevizos et al., (1978) was used for this purpose. The BOI consists of two types of behavioural categories: mutually exclusive behaviours and concomitant behaviours. All behaviours that can be observed in a given setting are categorised as one of the mutually exclusive behaviours, for example, sitting, standing, walking. These may be observed in conjunction with one or more of the concomitant behaviours, for example, talking, smoking, watching television, reading. For the purposes of the present study, it is the observation and classification of this latter category of behaviours which is significant, as it provides a measure of engagement and social activity. Alevizos et al., note that the methodology allows 'direct observation methods, once assumed by some to belong to the special province of the single subject design, (to be) used to assess the effect of programs on groups of psychiatric clients in an efficient and economic manner'.

It was determined that two observers would jointly conduct sweeps of the large building occupied by the ward, according to a predetermined plan, observing each individual present simultaneously for five seconds. These observational sweeps were taken between meal times, when patients had leisure time which might be used for recreational or social activity. A total of 525 observations was made, using coding classifications which had been determined by a pilot study. Only when every behaviour recorded in the five second interval agreed between observers was the observation scored as an agreement. The calculation of observer agreement in BOI observations used the method of percent effective agreement. This statistic is the ratio of mutually agreed occurrences. Agreement was calculated for the 525 individual five second observations. The percentage of effective agreement was 96%.

The resultant agreed observations are presented in Figure 3.5. They reflect a social environment in which there is a little stimulation for the patients. 45% of the observations found no concomitant behaviour at all, despite the fact that this was the very thing being looked for. In these observations, individuals were simply sitting or standing and not engaged in any way. Solitary activity, such as making tea alone, and solitary recreation such as watching television alone, account for another 25% of the observations. Inappropriate behaviours such as perseverative/unusual motor behaviour or perseverative/unusual verbal behaviour account for 16% of observations (for example, repeatedly swaying from side to side and repeated muttering or chanting to one's self). 2% of observations were of socially approved activities, such as washing pots or sweeping up. Only 12% of observations were accounted for by social interaction, both verbal and non-verbal, between patients, or patients and staff.

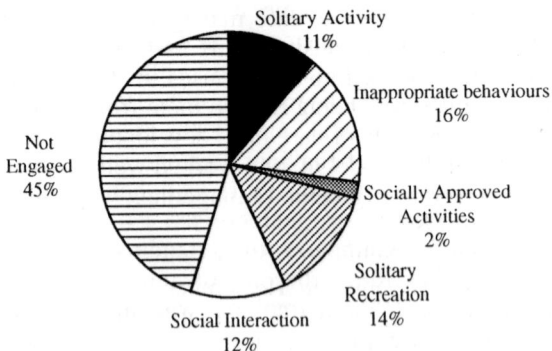

Figure 3.5
Hospital observation study: Concomitant behaviours

Low levels of staff - patient interaction in the old long-stay wards may be at least partially attributable to the lower staffing ratios on these wards. This in turn is an explanatory factor in the lower costs of care in these wards (chapter 7). Although levels of communication between staff and patients were observed to be low in old long-stay wards, nursing staff reported frequent discussion of patients' needs with fellow staff, some four-fifths having discussions daily. Such discussion, about patients, rather than with patients, is reflected in the comparatively low level of control which care staff attributed to patients in their daily lives. Patients had little choice in time of rising and taking meals, lacked variety of recreational activities and had little privacy, living communally and sleeping in dormitories. Patients were not involved in planning their own care programmes, although the desirability of patient involvement in the preparation of IAPs was recognised in the formal planning of resettlement procedures.

Few hospital nursing staff transferred to the community with patients they had cared for in hospital. The large majority of community staff were new appointments, mainly selected for qualities which involved personal characteristics or life experience. The mean age of community staff on appointment was thirty-nine years. The qualities which staff themselves most frequently mentioned as being important in their jobs revolved around their own life experiences. This 'normalisation' of care workers' perspectives, relating care to their own experience, rather than to any formal model of psychiatric care is a notable feature of residential care outside of the hospital setting. Community staff felt that residents had enhanced ease of access to community facilities. They perceived this as a method of normalisation which complemented and formed a part of IAPs.

The care manager, direct care staff and clients are all involved in daily decision making processes in Scheme I, where the care manager and deputy have an office in the group living scheme. In Scheme II, the care managers have less direct involvement in staff and client decision making. In this scheme staff perceive the care managers' role in terms of more costly expenditures, such as housing, staff and maintenance costs. The division of this care scheme into five houses in different locations has resulted in the care managers being more remote from every day decision making and devolved models of care have developed. In practice, staff in both schemes felt that the model of care worked well for clients, although a need was expressed for greater management support in the more dispersed residences of Scheme II.

Initial staff training in Scheme I consisted of a one week induction course. Subsequently individual staff member have been encouraged to attend a part-time training course in mental health care at Manchester University which is designed to enhance their professional skills. The course consists of modules which course members undertake on one day a week, leading to the Certificate of Mental Health Care. In Scheme II, induction consisted of a two week hospital-based course.

In the community IAPs have been based upon needs assessments by direct care workers and managers. These assessments have been made comprehensive and systematic in the care schemes. However, staff in the community care schemes also felt that a process of community integration was an important aspect of care management. Community care tends to be based on less formal concepts than hospital care management and direct care staff suggested 'responding to client wishes and needs', 'using my own life experience', 'undoing institutionalisation' and 'the method is common sense' as appropriate approaches to direct care, while managers suggested more formal methods such as 'role modelling, promoting everyday living skills' and 'a needs-led plan of care, an ongoing process based on strengths and needs'.

Multi-disciplinary assessment procedures in hospital are thorough and result in the preparation of IAPs. However, in the old long stay wards the implementation of plans and the involvement of clients in care programmes is frequently only partial. There has also been a tendency for the follow through of care plans from hospital to community to be incomplete. Good care planning requires a smooth follow through of plans from hospital to community. However, an important point to emerge was that support workers in Scheme II had had the opportunity to work in hospital prior to closure of the ward and moved to the community with their clients. Staff suggested that 'The process was very gradual for everyone.' 'You could find out about clients and ask questions'. 'It was very useful in getting to know the clients and them getting to know us.' This attitude was endorsed by one of the community care managers as a valuable part of the deinstitutionalisation process.

Both community care schemes have established procedures for regular review of care plans for individuals. Formal reviews take place on a six monthly basis in Scheme I, with informal reviews more frequently. In Scheme II there is a formal review for each team caring for three clients once a month. There has been a significant increase in the extent to which clients are involved in making decisions about their own lives and daily routine in the move from hospital to community. In the community the involvement of clients in decision-making is well exemplified by the full participation in their own reviews in Scheme I, which requires sensitive handling, but appears to be taken well by clients who contribute significantly to the discussion. It has information, participation and motivational advantages for clients and offers a means of developing self-awareness and self-confidence. This is illustrated in both case notes and IAPs (names have been changed):-

Malcolm used to make grunting noises and stand in corners. He would refuse to communicate and would sit for hours in the same position, staring blankly out of the window. Since moving to the community there has been a great improvement. He will talk and answer you. He is exceptionally clean and tidy. He now goes out more often to the shops and cafés and takes more interest in things around him. An important objective of his care plan is to draw him out further and to involve him in activities with other people.

Since moving into his new home Michael has played an active part in the domestic routine and appears to be settling in well. The sociable side of his personality has developed considerably. He is far less shy and will engage positively in conversation and he will make positive social gestures, such as offering tomatoes he has grown in the greenhouse. He frequently goes to the local shops alone, makes food and household purchases. Generally, he appears to have benefited considerably from the move to the community which has enabled him to overcome much of his withdrawn behaviour and has developed his potential for positive social behaviours.

Greater involvement in decision-making and responsibility for making choices is seen as an important part of care management in the community. Increased personal responsibility is seen as an important part of the process by 61% of community staff. Developing increased confidence (44%) and mixing in the community (39%) were also seen as important elements in a developing care process. These aspects of care are not easy developments for all residents and staff felt that some 50% of clients would find difficulty in developing in these directions. Because the assessment of individual needs by keyworkers forms an important part of forming IAPs and implementing care management in the community, it was decided to undertake a formal assessment of client needs with keyworkers in Scheme I and Scheme II.

An assessment instrument for use with keyworkers was developed, based on the Personal Social Services Research Unit's Case Review Assessment (PSSRU, 1986), which assesses an individual's need for care and need for services. The overall system provides a normative, service led orientation to need, which provides a systematic approach to the classification and quantification of need. Following a pilot study with keyworkers, need was classified in social, functional and clinical categories and the degree of need for individuals was measured in each dimension by the extent to which support was considered necessary by the keyworker. The extent to which each dimension of need was considered to be met, was also assessed, ranging from unmet, through partially met to fully met. Assessments were undertaken with a keyworker for each resident after twelve months community residence, giving a total of 24 assessments for the residents of Community Scheme I and Community Scheme II. The results for the extent of need perceived in each area by keyworkers are presented in Figure 3.6.

The greatest client needs perceived by managers and workers were domestic, financial and accommodation. Key workers focus on these basic needs and place less emphasis on areas in where it may be more difficult to work, such as developing social skills, personal care, occupational activities and mental health care needs. The low level of mental health care need perceived by staff is surprising in schemes which have continuing medical supervision by consultant psychiatrists and community psychiatric nurses, and in which maintenance of medication is seen as an essential contribution to the stabilisation of psychiatric symptoms. The enhanced social component of care in the community may provide an explanation. The two care schemes are generally seen by staff to offer a comprehensive care service to clients in which other services such as primary health care teams and consultant psychiatrist make important contributions to a more holistic pattern of care. However, low levels of perceived mental health care need are not fully consistent with research data showing the prevalence of psychiatric symptomatology (chapter 4) and the recognition by staff that they require training in the management of difficult and aggressive behaviours.

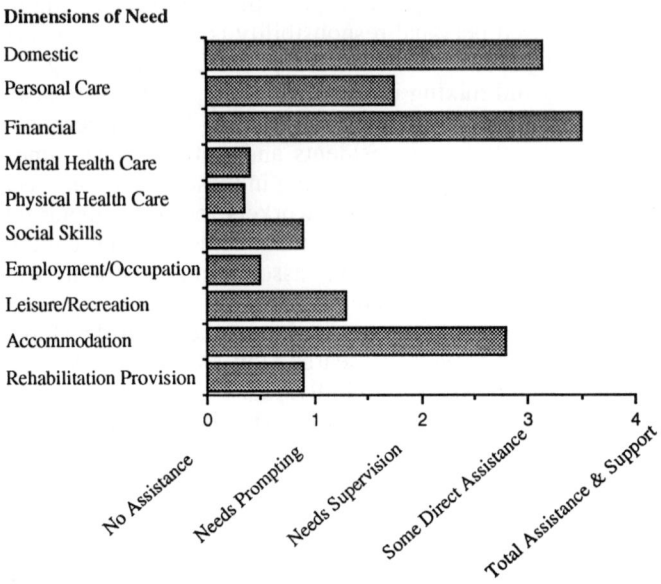

Figure 3.6
Keyworker assessment of clients' needs

The survey of clients' needs with key workers and managers indicated that they generally considered a high proportion of perceived need to be met by the care packages provided. This was particularly the case with domestic, financial, recreational and accommodation needs. In other words, needs that are recognised by managers and key workers are felt to be met to a high degree. The extent to which care workers in the community are succeeding in modifying behaviour patterns is reflected in the following case review comments:-

When Ralph first came to community care he was very unsure of himself and appeared to revert to the 'psychiatric patient role' to get his own way over such things as having cigarettes and avoiding baths and getting up in the morning, or doing certain chores for himself. He appeared in these early days to be very insecure and institutionalised. However, over the past 6 months he has made great inroads in diminishing some of these problems. At first there were tantrums of verbal aggression in the order of twice or three times a day.

However, with his new-found confidence these have reduced to something in the order of perhaps two or three per month. Lack of cigarettes is now the most common trigger for these occasional outbursts, but overall he has done very well in this area. He still needs prompting and support with laundry, shopping and budgeting. Overall, although there are some areas which need considerable staff support, he has settled happily and has made considerable improvements in his social and behavioural functioning.

Staff attitudes in the hospital and community settings

A total of sixty-nine staff were interviewed using the Staff Attitudes and Management Practices schedule. Formal documentation such as philosophies of care, care programmes and case records were also inspected as a basis against which to interpret staff attitudes to care.Thirty-three staff were hospital based and thirty six were community based. Hospital based staff were selected from the long-stay and rehabilitation wards from which patients in the research cohort were expected to be discharged to care in the community. 60% of the hospital staff were qualified psychiatric nurses and 40% were nursing assistants. Community based staff included all managers and support workers who provided the care and support in the two community residential schemes into which the majority of those resettled from the hospital were discharged. The mean age of the community residential care staff was 39 years. 83% had previous care related experience, which was useful in that they has some insight into mental health problems and importantly, they had had previous contact with people who had experienced mental health problems. 19% had qualifications in the psychiatric nursing/caring professions.

For the purpose of this study, data from the community-based residential care schemes were combined. The reason for this was that the main focus of the study was to compare staff attitudes in hospital with those of care staff in the community. Where comparisons are thought to be important between the two community schemes, these will be discussed.

Staff attitudes to resettlement

Hospital. A majority of hospital staff were positive about the changing nature of their job. 60% of hospital staff reported feeling prepared for change in their job. A similar proportion of staff (56%) had chosen to work on rehabilitation. When asked whether or not there was anything they would like to see changed 76% of the replies concerned issues related to a lack of information with regard to the hospital closure and job security. Staff wanted: 'More cooperation between management and staff'. 'Reversal of the hospital closure'. 'Like to know what is happening'. 'There is uncertainty, dissatisfaction with not knowing what's going to happen to the residents'. It is interesting to note that many hospital staff apparently distinguished between the merit of the policy of community care and their future job security. The majority of hospital staff perceived a move to community-based care for their clients positively. 63% described themselves as pleased with the impending move, while 25% were 'not at all pleased' with the move. The finding that one-quarter of those interviewed were so displeased was associated with those staff having negative attitudes to their clients' prospects in the community, and hospital staff expressing dissatisfaction with their job security. The hospital staff were polarised and hospital managers experienced considerable difficulty in dealing with the disaffected group.

Community. After twelve months in the community, the process of resettlement was felt to be successful by 89% of the community care staff. A large number of positive comments were made by community staff: 'It's beyond what I expected, especially with older clients'. 'Two here did not want to move, seeing them settle is great'. 'Just seeing differences in the clients and having visitors notice is rewarding'. 'They have a better way of life now'. 'They like being here and do not want to go back to hospital'. 'They get to do things they would not been able to do in hospital'. 'Greater freedom and choice'. The high level of perceived success in the early stages of community care may be tempered in the future but it does indicate the positive commitment of staff to the care schemes in which they were working. Community staff felt that now clients were in the community care setting, access to and the ease with which community facilities could be utilised increased the opportunity of 'mixing with the public'. They perceived it as a method of normalisation which enhanced formal client programmes.

Employment satisfaction

Hospital. A high proportion (88%) of the hospital staff expressed general satisfaction in relation to their work. Examples of what hospital staff were satisfied with included:- 83% being satisfied with their own accomplishments, and 73% being satisfied with the management and supervision given by their superiors. (See Figure 3.7). However, there were causes for dissatisfaction: 62% were dissatisfied with opportunities for advancement within the service and 39% expressed dissatisfaction about job security. In response to open-ended questioning, the main problems identified by the hospital staff concerned the anticipated hospital closure and the perception that management were not providing information about policy decisions. 'Somebody knows... why don't they come out with it'. 'There should be a programme of preparation'. 'There is no opportunity to discuss my future or the future of the patients'.

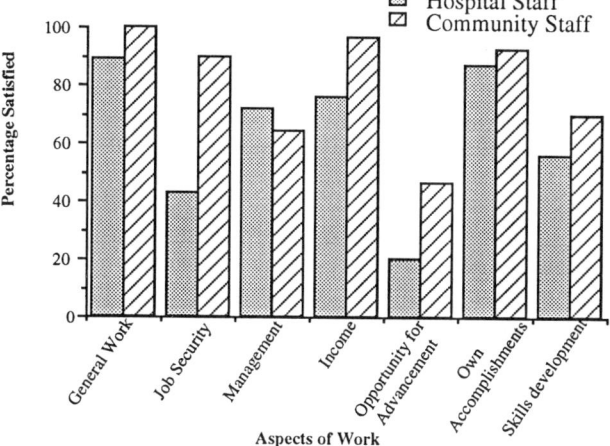

Figure 3.7
Expressed satisfaction levels of hospital and community care staff

Community. All community staff reported being either 'very' or 'quite' satisfied with their work. Very high levels of job satisfaction were reported by community staff in terms the flexibility of the hours worked (100%), opportunities to use their own initiative (100%), income (97%), relationships with fellow workers (95%), number of hours worked (95%), ease of travel to work (92%), the actual tasks done (89%) and job security (70%). Areas of dissatisfaction included opportunities for advancement within the service. 47% of the staff in Community Scheme II indicated dissatisfaction with this item as opposed to 75% of the staff in Scheme I who found such opportunities to be satisfactory.

Although community workers are generally satisfied with their job there were some negative attitudes toward how they saw their career developing. In Scheme II, the initial enthusiasm for a new project and the difficulty of maintaining that enthusiasm, particularly when caring for an older group of clients, made some staff feel that in the future they would leave the scheme and perhaps join a scheme with younger clients.

Staff concerns

Hospital. Although 73% of the hospital staff reported being satisfied with management and supervision by their superiors, and 88% reported general approval in terms of job satisfaction, the analysis suggests dissatisfaction with the hospital closure in terms of the potential loss of jobs on the one hand and concern about the reality of care in the community on the other. This can be related to hospital staff having reservations about community residential care being bad for those discharged from hospital. When asked to describe the worst possible outcome of resettlement 75% of the hospital staff feared the worst outcome would be reduced care levels for the clients, 12% feared 'failure outside', and 9% feared 'public resentment'.

Community. Developing client-centred programmes of care and a needs-led service involves responding flexibly to clients whose behaviour can present challenges to managers and direct care workers. In hospital, staff had not reported experiencing client-centred problems but in the community 26% of staff found difficulties of this kind. Frustration and stress with difficult clients are reported, as is difficulty in dealing with mood swings. Skilled managerial support is essential for staff in these circumstances and there is also a strong demand for further training by staff. 83% of Scheme II staff felt that further training and qualifications were necessary to provide care effectively. The need for staff training mainly related to providing greater insight into mental illness and the management of challenging behaviour.

Discussion

This chapter has examined the socially relevant physical characteristics, care practices and staff attitudes of the hospital and two main community settings in which the psychiatric, behavioural and quality of life outcomes were investigated for members of the research cohort. It is clear that the resettlement of patients to better physical environments gave greater opportunity for privacy, personalisation, independence and access to community facilities. These considerations are relevant to a process of normalisation, in which the physical environment has a role to play in providing an opportunity and supportive setting for community orientated care. In hospital, all four wards studied afforded comparatively poor or constricting facilities in which to conduct the care of psychiatric patients. The community settings provide much more appropriate environments for care programmes directed to normalisation, and, coupled with new, less restrictive care regimes, offer the opportunity for creative work, which one would expect to be reflected in the measures of outcome for those in the research group.

Care management tends to place emphasis on the assessment of the individual client and the coordination of care through an agreed individual action plan. Elements of both case management and care management models are present in the management and delivery of care in community Schemes I and II. This combination of models is important because it demonstrates how hybrid care patterns tend to develop in the provision of community care. It is also important to note that both schemes offer that integration of care provision which has been described as 'seamless' delivery of services. This is the recognised aim of formal case management models. At the same time, the lack of integration of service provision for those patients resettled from hospital to living alone or to some family situations, with a range of fragmented services - social work, community psychiatric nursing, day hospital, consultant appointments - is an example of the difficulties besetting community care which care management is intended to overcome.

It is clear that in the establishment of the two community schemes considered here, the pursuit of particular models of management was less important than the concern of the professionals involved to provide integrated care to meet the needs of particular client groups. Thus, both Schemes I and II were established with management involvement in care delivery as well as workers with key worker and care management roles. This blurring of distinctions between role models does not sit easily with case management models, but it has provided effective care delivery.

An account has been provided of hospital care and the differences between this and two new community settings to which clients have been relocated. The assumptions of environmental determinism have been balanced by an analysis of care practices and staff attitudes in both old and new settings, which suggests that substantial changes have taken place, leading to enhanced client participation in the formulation of objectives and care practices. The focus of this process takes full advantage of the new location of care settings and the domestic character of environments. The assessment of need is part of the process of formulating care plans or individual action plans. The development and implementation of IAPs is the basis of individual care management and of ensuring the quality of that care in both hospital and community. In hospital IAPs were developed by multidisciplinary teams but it was rare for clients to participate directly in this process. In hospital very little decision-making involved clients. Staff reported that no patients were involved in deciding about their programmes of care, although 'contracts' were made with patients to try to establish behavioural standards. The two community schemes represent a pattern of care provision which is informed by the re-development of concepts of psychiatric care. Each emphasises domesticity, rather than institutionalism, each focuses upon individual needs and seeks a means of realising these through individual action plans, which target community participation and responsibility for, and control of, ones own life. The critical test of the efficacy of these new approaches lies in the results of outcome measures which form the central part of this study.

References

Alevizos, P., DeRisi, W., Liberman, R., Eckman, T. and Callahan, E. (1978), 'The Behaviour Observation Instrument: A Method of Direct Observation for Program Evaluation', *Journal of Applied Behaviour Analysis*, 2, 243-257.

Appleyard, D. (1979), 'Home', *Architectural Association Quarterly,* 2, 2-20.

Barton, R. (1959), *Institutional Neurosis.* Bristol, John Wright and Sons Ltd.

Becker, F. (1973), *Housing Messages.* Stoudsberg PA: Dowden Hutchinson and Ross.

Becker, H.S. (1963) *,Outsiders,* New York, The Free Press.

Booth, T. (1985), *Home Truths: Old People's Homes and the Outcome of Care.* Aldershot: Gower.

Clough, R. (1981), *Old Age Homes.* London: George Allen and Unwin.

Clwyd Health Authority (1991), *Clwyd Plan for Mental Illness Services.* Clwyd Health Authority, Mold, North Wales.

Cooper, C. (1972), 'The house as a symbol of self', *Design and Environment,* 3, 30-37.

Cooper, C. (1974), 'The house as a symbol of the self' in J. T. Long (ed), *Designing for Human Behaviour.* Stroudsberg, Penn: Dowden Hutchinson and Ross.

Copeland, J.R.M., Crosby, C., Sixsmith, J.A. and Stillwell, J. (1988), 'District Experimental Care Schemes', *Interim Report.* Department of Psychiatry/Institute of Human Ageing, Liverpool University.

DHSS (1981), *Growing Older,* Cmnd 8173. London: HMSO.

Duncan, J.S. and Duncan, N.G. (1976a), 'Housing as presentation of self and the structure of social networks', in G.T. Moore and R. College (eds), *Enviromental Knowing: Theories Research and Methods.* Stoudsberg, Penn: Dowden, Hutchinson and Ross.

Duncan, J.S. and Duncan, N.G.(1976b), 'Social worlds, status passage and environmental persepectives', in G.T. Moore and R. College (eds), *Enviromental Knowing: Theories Research and Methods.* Stroudsberg: Dowden, Hutchinson and Ross.

Erikson, E.H. (1968), *Identity: Youth and Crisis.* New York: Norton.

Fisk, M.J. (1987), *Independence and the Elderly,* London. Croom Helm.

Ford, R., Repper, J., Cooke, A., Norton, P., Beadsmore, A. and Clark, C. (1993), 'Implementing Case Management', *Research and Development for Psychiatry.* London.

Garety, P.A. and Morris, I. (1984), 'A new unit for long-stay psychiatric patients: Organisation, attitudes and quality of life', *Psychological Medicine,* 14, 183-192.

Goffman, E. (1959), *Presenting of Self in Everyday Life.* New York: Doubleday.

Goffman, E. (1968), 'Asylums: Essays on the Social Situation of Mental Patients and Other Inmates'. New York. Anchor Books, Doubleday & Co (reprint 1961).

Gurney, C. and Means, R. (1993), 'The meaning of home in later life', in S. Arber and M. Evandrou (eds), *Ageing, Independence and the Life Course*, 119-31. London. Jessica Kingsley.

Harrison, L. and Means, R. (1990), *Housing: The Essential Element in Community Care.* London:SHAC and Anchor Housing Trust.

Hayward, D.G. (1977), 'Home as an environmental and psychological concept', *Landscape,* 20 (1) 2-9.

Higgins, J. (1989), 'Defining community care: realisties and myths', *Social Policy and Administration,* Vol. 23, 1, 3-16.

Jones, K. (1988), *Experience in Mental Health, Community Care and Social Policy.* London. Sage Publications.

Lemert, E. (1951), *Social Pathology.* New York. The Free Press.

Meacher, M. (1969), 'The future of community care', in J. Agate and M. Meacher (eds) *The Care of the Old.* London: Fabian Society.

Means, R. and Smith, R. (1994), *Community Care: Policy and Practice.* MacMillan, London.

Munnichs, J. (1976) 'Dependency, interdependence and autonomy', in J. Munnichs and J. Van der Heuval (eds), *Dependency and Interdependency in Old Age.* The Hague: Martinus Nijhoff.

Murphy, E. (1991), *After the Asylums: Community Care for People with Mental Illness.* London. Faber and Faber.

Personal Social Services Research Unit. (1986), *Care in the Community Initiative: Guide to the Evaluation.* PSSRU. University of Kent at Canterbury.

Pratt, G. (1982), 'The house as an expression of social worlds', in J.S Duncan (eds) *Housing and Identity.* New York: Homes and Meier.

Rapoport, A. (1969) *House Form and Culture.* New Jersey: Prentice-Hall.

Rapoport, A. (1982), *The Meaning of the Built Environment*. London: Sage.

Richardson, A. (1977), 'Organisation and Interaction of Psychatric Day Centres'. Unpublished M. Phil Dissertation. University of London.

Robinson, J.W., Thompson T., Emmons P., and Graff M. (1984), *Towards an Architectural Definition of Normalisation*. School of Architecture, University of Minnesota.

Rotegard, L.L, Bruninks, R.H. and Hill, B.K., (1981), *Environmental Charactersistics of Residential Facilities for Mentally Retarded People*. Minneapolis, MN: University of Minesota.

Ryan, P., Ford, R, and Clifford, P. (1991), *Case Management and Community Care*. Research and Development for Psychiatry.

Scull, A.T. (1979), *Museums of Madness: The Social Organisation of Insanity in Nineteenth Centry England*. London, Penguin Books.

Scull, A.T. (1984), Decarceration: Community Treatment and the Deviant. *A Radical View*. Cambridge Press.

Sixsmith, J. (1986), 'The meaning of home: an exporatory study of environmental experience', *Journal of Environmental Psychology*, 6, 281-298.

Steinfield, E. (1981), 'The place of old age', in J.S. Duncan (ed), *Housing and Identity*. New York: Holmes and Meier.

Tobin, S.S. and M.A. Lieberman (1976), *Last Home for the Aged*. San Francisco: Jossey-Bass.

Townsend, P. (1962), *The Last Refuge*. London: Routledge and Kegan Paul.

Willcocks, D., Pearce S. and Kellaher L. (1987), *Private Lives in Public Places*. London: Tavistock.

Wing, J.K. (ed) (1982), 'Long term Community Care: Experience in a London Borough, *Psychological Medicine*. Monography Supplement 2.

Wykes, T. (1982), 'A hostel ward for 'new' long-stay patients: An evaluative study of a 'ward in a house''. *In Long-Term Community Care: Experience in a London Borough*. (ed. J.K. Wing), pp. 57-97. Psychological Medicine Monograph Supplement 2.

4 Psychiatric and behavioural outcomes for clients twelve months after discharge from hospital

Charles Crosby, Margaret M.Barry and Susan A. Geertshuis

Summary

In this chapter the analysis of the psychiatric and behavioural outcome measures is presented. The process of change over time is considered. By 12 months post-discharge, 34 clients had been resettled from hospital to community settings; 31 patients had remained in hospital. For those resettled, the results show that psychiatric state has tended to remain stable in the post-discharge period, with some significant improvements in individual indices, in particular in a lessening of blunted affect and emotional withdrawal. For the resettlement group as a whole, there have been significant improvements in social and behavioural functioning. The results are also presented for two main sub-groups, one group comprised of 'new long-stay' patients, the other 'old long-stay' patients. Psychiatric characteristics measured at hospital baseline have persisted through to the twelve months post-discharge assessment for both groups. There have been significant gains for the 'old long-stay' group in social functioning which has lessened the initial difference between the two groups in this respect. The outcomes for both client groups are shown to be related to the environmental and care practice characteristics of the two care schemes to which they have been allocated. The results indicate that continuing high levels of supportive professional care and social care are needed for those resettled from hospital to community. Given this support individuals may attain higher levels of functioning and enhanced freedom and independence.

Introduction

This chapter is intended to provide analysis of the data gathered in accordance with the research procedures discussed in chapter 2. The objective of the study is to implement a comprehensive series of psychiatric and behavioural assessments with a cohort of patients resident in hospital who were expected to be resettled to a variety of community care settings in the course of the evaluation study. The stability of the results of the three baseline assessment points in hospital strengthens the predictive nature of the study, which anticipates that changes in care environments and care practices will be reflected in the outcome measures. The strength of the research design and the potential validity of an interrupted times series with replications have been established in chapter 2. The design of this study bears similarities to that used in the study of outcomes of resettlement by the Team for the Assessment of Psychiatric Services (TAPs, Anderson et al., 1993). The design of the TAPs study is naturalistic, rather than experimental. A randomised study was not considered to be possible because the movement out of hospital depended on the capacity of the different resettlement districts to find care provision in the community. Those patients who were defined as long-stay by an admission of more than one year and a diagnosis other than senile dementia were included in the study. Baseline hospital assessments were then undertaken, and when a patient was due to be discharged a suitable matched patient was identified. The mover and the 'match' were then reinterviewed 12 months after the mover's discharge. The TAPs assessments include a mental state examination, an assessment of social and behavioural functioning, a patient attitude questionnaire, an environmental index, and a social network schedule. After the first three years of the TAPs study it was concluded that all the clear differences in outcomes over time indicated advantages for the discharged patients. Those who left hospital were living lives which were less restrictive than the 'matches' in hospital experienced. Reflecting this, leavers changed markedly in their first year in the community, to show more positive attitudes towards their care environments and treatment. However, the findings concerning clinical outcomes were more equivocal. There were some minor increases in psychiatric symptomatology for hospital leavers. It is concluded that not only were the long-stay patients discharged to the community living under much less restrictive conditions than in hospital, but they also greatly preferred life in the community and were appreciative of their new homes. Their mental state and social disabilities were stable, but they had made new friends who were drawn from ordinary members of the community.

The work undertaken by the TAPs project has demonstrated that there are positive benefits for clients resettled to well resourced community schemes.

The longitudinal repeated measures design of the present study is similar to that used in the TAPs project. The research design provides for the continuing assessment of those who remain in hospital at twelve monthly intervals after the initial hospital baseline assessments. This has facilitated comparison with the clients who have been resettled to the community. Thus the whole research cohort has continued to be assessed, whether located in hospital or community.

The importance of studies which monitor psychiatric outcomes should be stressed. Such studies provide a scientific basis on which the evaluation of changes in social policy with regard to the care of psychiatric populations may be monitored. The research is designed to monitor changes in mental state, social and behavioural functioning and quality of life (Crosby et al., 1993).

The research instruments have been fully described in chapter 2. They include; The Brief Psychiatric Rating Scale (BPRS; Overall and Gorham, 1962), The Scale for the Assessment of Negative Symptoms (SANS-AF., Andreason, 1982, and The Krawiecka Rating Scale (KRS; Krawiecka et al., 1977), The Rehabilitation Evaluation of Hall and Baker (REHAB; Baker and Hall, 1983). Repeated measures analysis (MANOVA) was carried out on each of the outcome measures, comparing the hospital baseline findings for discharged patients with levels of functioning at 12 months post-discharge. Similar analyses were undertaken for those remaining in hospital, comparing later assessments with the three initial baseline assessments. Thus each client served as their own control in the study, permitting a direct comparison of levels of functioning in the hospital and community care settings, before and after discharge.

Sample characteristics

The analysis of the hospital baseline and subsequent hospital assessments has shown that there were two main groupings of clients in the present study - 'old long-stay' clients who had spent many years in hospital, and 'new long-stay' clients, for whom a similar lifetime career in psychiatric hospital would be predicted if there had not been changes in national policy and in the implementation of the All-Wales Mental Health Strategy in North Wales - (Welsh Office, 1989; Clwyd Health Authority, 1991). It is important to note that there were no initial significant differences in the three hospital assessments between those who remained in hospital and those resettled with regard to age, length of hospitalisation, mental state, deviant behaviour and social and behavioural functioning. However, there was a well defined process of assessment and selection for resettlement by the multidisplinary teams in the 'new long-stay' wards which resulted in the selection of individuals who were considered more likely to succeed in community care settings. This process involved self selection to a limited degree, in that those who were positively motivated towards leaving the hospital were more likely to be considered to have good prospects of successfully settling in new locations.

All individuals included in the cohort had been in hospital continuously for more than one year. The initial distinction between Community Scheme 1 and Community Scheme II residents is evident when the data are reviewed for each establishment (see chapter 3 for a description of these community schemes). In Scheme I the mean length of life time hospitalisation had been 16.4 years (SD 13.4), while the mean age was 48 years (SD 8.1). In Scheme II the mean lifetime hospitalisation was 32.7 years (SD 8.3) and mean age was 66 years (SD 6.6). The resettlement process provided specialist care for two distinct client groups with clearly defined characteristics in two main community care schemes. These differences extend further, to include psychiatric symptomatology and social and behavioural functioning. The analysis of the BPRS results shows that in the hospital assessments, those who were to be residents in Scheme I had higher levels of active psychiatric symptomatology than those who were to be resident in Scheme II. The results of hospital assessments show that Scheme I residents were also characterised initially by a lower mean total general behaviour score in the REHAB assessments (indicating lower levels of behavioural impairment) than those patients who were to move to Scheme II. One may therefore conclude that these two groups typically represented the 'new long-stay' and 'old long-stay' psychiatric patients described in chapter 2, prior to resettlement in the new community based care establishments.

Outcomes for the entire resettlement group

Once clients had been resettled from hospital to the community, research assessments took place at 6 weeks, 6 months and twelve months post-discharge to monitor the process of adjustment to new environments and patterns of care. There were 29 respondents in the community sample at 12 months post-discharge. At the corresponding hospital assessment there were 26 respondents. Three respondents had died of natural causes in each group. Two members of the community group refused to participate in the twelve months post-discharge assessments and two in the hospital groups were not interviewable due to acute psychiatric problems. Eleven of those who had initially remained in hospital had been resettled to the community, but had not yet reached the 12 months post-discharge assessment point. There had also been short-term hospital readmissions for the two members of the community sample who had been resettled to independent living, in each case to socially and physically isolated locations. The results of the mental state assessments will be considered first.

The three-monthly repeated assessments while in hospital were examined for those who were discharged. These show no significant variations while patients remained in hospital. Following resettlement, levels of psychiatric symptomatology as measured by the BPRS, KRS and SANS-AF showed a number of significant changes from those measures at hospital baseline.

Table 4.1

Brief Psychiatric Rating Scale (BPRS) Mean item scores; hospital baseline, 6 weeks, 6 months and 12 months post-discharge (N=29)

Factor Scores	Hospital Baseline		6 weeks Post-discharge		6 months Post-discharge		12 months Post-discharge		Baseline/ 12 months Post-discharge
	M	(SD)	M	(SD)	M	(SD)	M	(SD)	F Ratio
Anxiety- Depression	.77	(1.06)	.69	(.74)	.75	(.72)	.99	(1.18)	.82
Anergia	.66	(1.12)	.45	(.61)	.34	(.70)	.27	(.51)	3.96*
Thought Disorder	1.16	(1.43)	1.23	(1.52)	1.10	(1.60)	1.23	(1.73)	.06
Activation	.73	(.81)	.69	(.63)	.78	(.83)	.90	(.97)	.34
Hostility-Suspiciousness	.51	(76)	.79	(.94)	.71	(.81)	1.01	(1.21)	4.70**
BPRS Total Scores	12.64	(12.79)	12.85	(10.25)	14.03	(14.31)	11.89	(9.98)	.02

Significance * P < 0.05; ** P < 0.01

The BPRS factor scores were analysed with significant changes emerging in relation to two of the factors. The anergia factor (comprising emotional withdrawal, motor retardation and blunted affect) shows a significant decrease (F=3.96, P<0.05) after 1 year in the community, and the hostility-suspiciousness factor (comprising hostility, suspiciousness and uncooperativeness) shows a significant increase (F=4.70, P<0.01) over baseline. The decrease in the anergia score continues from 6 weeks post-discharge through 6 months down to its 12 months post-discharge level. The increase in the hostility-suspiciousness factor score is less even (Table 4.1). The BPRS total score shows no significant change between hospital baseline and 12 months post-discharge, although there is some temporary increase at the 6 month point. The mean scores for individual item ratings show only two significant changes from baseline to 12 months post-discharge; a decrease in blunted affect (F= 4.48, P<0.05) and a decrease in emotional withdrawal (F= 4.08, P=0.05).

These findings are consistent with those observed in relation to the SANS-AF. A significant reduction in negative symptoms was found in relation to two of the items rated on the SANS-AF; facial expression (F=12.18, P<0.01) and spontaneous movements (F=4.67, P<0.05) Table 4.2. The KRS results show significant changes in the mean score for depression with the 12 months post-discharge data showing a significant reduction in depression levels (F= 4.91, P<0.05) Table 4.3.

Table 4.2
Scale for the Assessment of Negative Symptoms (SANS-AF) Mean item scores; hospital baseline, 6 weeks, 6 months and 12 months post-discharge (N=29)

	Hospital Baseline		6 weeks Post-discharge		6 months Post-discharge		12 months Post-discharge		Baseline/ 12 months Post-discharge
	M	(SD)	M	(SD)	M	(SD)	M	(SD)	F Ratio
Facial Expression	1.14	(1.39)	.56	(.86)	.29	(.91)	.15	(.45)	12.18**
Spontaneous Movement	.55	(1.18)	.33	(.72)	.17	(64)	.04	(.20)	4.67*
Expressive Gestures	.73	(1.39)	.40	(.70)	.31	(.75)	.17	(.58)	3.48
Eye Contact	.62	(1.28)	.48	(.88)	.46	(.91)	.40	(1.11)	.36
Affectivity	.46	(1.14)	.42	(.76)	.08	(.32)	.17	(.48)	.88
Vocal Inflection	.48	(.75)	.40	(.62)	.48	(1.05)	.31	(.82)	.21

Significance * P < 0.05; ** P< 0.01

Table 4.3
Krawiecka Rating Scale (KRS) Mean item scores; hospital baseline, 6 weeks, 6 months and 12 months post-discharge (N=29)

	Hospital Baseline		6 weeks Post-discharge		6 months Post-discharge		12 months Post-discharge		Baseline/ 12 months Post-discharge
Ratings based on verbal report									
	M	(SD)	M	(SD)	M	(SD)	M	(SD)	F Ratio
Depressed	0.60	(1.03)	0.43	(.55)	0.33	(0.56)	0.29	(.78)	4.91*
Anxious	0.88	(.96)	1.05	(.95)	1.07	(1.00)	1.13	(1.16)	1.68
Coherent delusions	1.22	(1.68)	1.35	(1.68)	0.93	(1.62)	1.29	(1.88)	0.05
Hallucinations	0.90	(1.61)	0.38	(.93)	0.4	(1.23)	0.92	(1.65)	0.01
Ratings based on behaviour during interview									
Incoherence of speech	0.65	(1.07)	0.3	(.84)	0.74	(1.30)	0.87	(1.42)	0.51
Poverty of speech	0.61	(1.07)	0.71	(.83)	0.64	(1.15)	0.59	(.91)	0.02
Flattened, incongruous affect	0.64	(.97)	0.79	(.75)	0.3	(.81)	0.52	(.85)	0.42
Psychomotor retardation	0.45	(.77)	0.38	(.52)	0.41	(.86)	0.27	(.57)	2.39

Significance: *P<0.05

These results indicate that after 12 months community living there has been no general deterioration in mental state and some evidence of improvement in specific areas. Rather, there has been a tendency for stability and continuity in the results of the psychiatric assessments. The changes which have occurred may be related to the increased stimulation and pressures of community living and tend to suggest increased awareness and liveliness in respondents, coupled with increased hostility and suspicion in the face of the changed environments and care practices which are being experienced. This is not surprising in view of the fact that few changes in type or dosage of medication took place in the first twelve months post-hospital discharge. Medical supervision continued through consultant out-patient appointments, community psychiatric nurses and primary health care teams. For the large majority who moved to supervised care situations, care workers assumed responsibility for ensuring compliance with medication.

Social and behavioural functioning

The analysis of the REHAB data indicates greater changes in social and behavioural functioning than were observed in the psychiatric assessments. There is a significant reduction in the REHAB total general behaviour score post-discharge which moves from a mean of 58.11 (SD 32.12) in hospital to 46.67 (SD 24.80) in the community (F6.62, P<0.01) indicating improved social and behavioural functioning. (Table 4.4)

Table 4.4
Hall & Baker REHAB
Mean factor scores; hospital baseline, 6 weeks, 6 months and 12 months post-discharge (N=29)

Factors	Hospital Baseline M	(SD)	6 weeks Post-discharge M	(SD)	6 months Post-discharge M	(SD)	12 months Post-discharge M	(SD)	Baseline/ 12 months Post-discharge F Ratio
Social Activity	24.55	(14.53)	18.23	(12.32)	15.64	(11.89)	17.88	(11.10)	7.75**
Speech Skills	6.69	(5.25)	4.35	(3.98)	4.37	(4.23)	4.13	(3.93)	9.18**
Disturbed Speech	4.76	(4.19)	3.73	(2.76)	3.81	(3.56)	4.02	(3.35)	2.09
Self Care	14.81	(11.61)	11.89	(9.94)	12.09	(10.09)	13.33	(8.54)	.48
Community Skills	9.50	(6.12)	7.09	(5.17)	6.76	(4.76)	6.68	(4.73)	6.92**
Total General Behaviour	58.11	(32.12)	44.23	(25.37)	42.09	(26.59)	46.67	(24.80)	6.62**
Total Deviant Behaviour	1.34	(1.19)	1.38	(1.57)	1.52	(1.65)	1.59	(1.83)	.30

Significance   ** P<0.01

The REHAB provides clinical judgements alongside the total general behaviour score ratings. These results show an improvement in the clinical judgements from 'could only live out (of hospital) if supervised' to 'borderline potential for living out (of hospital). Needs extensive training and experience first' (Baker and Hall, 1985).

Levels of deviant behaviour measured by the REHAB show no significant change from hospital to 12 months post-discharge. The main improvement in the total general behaviour score is observed at 6 weeks post-discharge, with further slight improvement at 6 months and a slight deterioration at 12 months (Fig 4.1). This suggests that, following an initial period of rapid improvement, a levelling off is occurring.

Inspection of the REHAB factor scores also reveals significant improvements from hospital baseline to twelve months post-discharge. With regard to the factor scores, significant improvements were found for levels of social activity (F=7.75, P<0.01), speech (F=9.18, P<0.01) and community skills (F= 6.62, P<0.01).

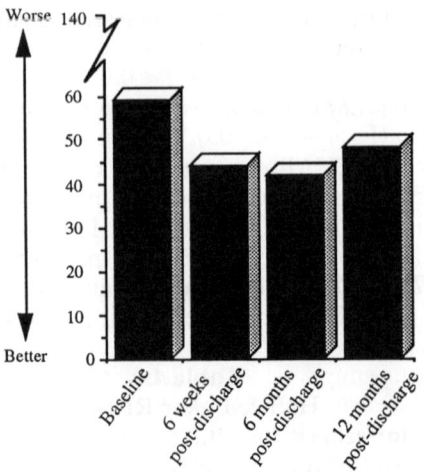

Figure 4.1
**REHAB Mean total general behaviour score. Hospital baseline, 6
weeks, 6 months and 12 months post-discharge (N=29)**

These results indicate increased social participation following discharge
from hospital. These improvements were evident at the 6 weeks post-
discharge assessment point and have continued to the 12 month post-
discharge assessment. Such improved factor scores are the main elements
contributing to the improved total general behavioural score. Changes in
factor scores are shown in Figure 4.2.

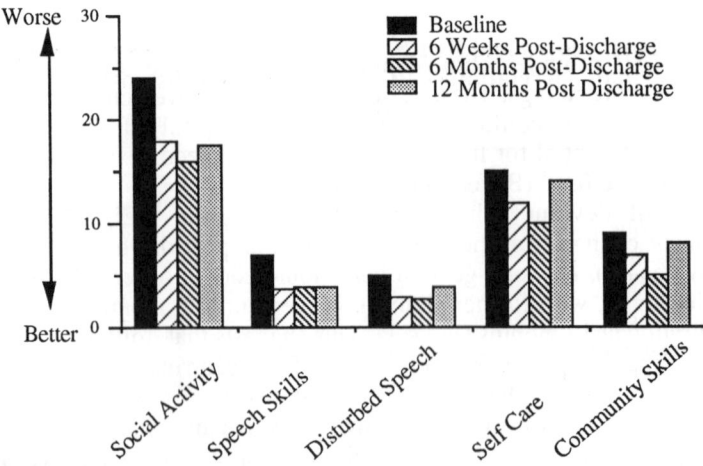

Figure 4.2
**REHAB Mean factor scores; Hospital baseline, 6 weeks, 6 months
post-discharge (N=29)**

A number of significant improvements were found in relation to the individual REHAB items. Clients were rated as exhibiting higher levels of mixing in the care setting ($F= 5.09$, $P< 0.05$) and out of the care setting ($F= 6.68$, $P<0.01$); they also showed improvements in relation to the amount of speech ($F=5.74$, $P<0.05$), the sense of the speech used ($F=5.91$, $P<0.05$) and the degree to which they initiated speech ($F=9.17$, $P<0.01$). A significant increase in the use of public facilities was also rated ($F=9.35$, $P<0.01$).

Mental state and social and behavioural functioning

The improvement in the BPRS Total Score and Anergia Factor Score suggested that these might be associated with the increased social activity, improvement in speech skills and community skills and enhanced self care levels noted in the REHAB results. Spearman Correlation Coefficients for the resettlement groups were therefore obtained. At twelve months post-discharge there are a number of significant correlations between the REHAB factor scores, total general behaviour score and the BPRS anergia factor and BPRS total score. These are presented in Table 4.5. Strong positive correlations exist between social activity and anergia and the BPRS total score. Speech skills correlate positively with anergia and self care has a significant positive correlation with the BPRS total score. Finally, the REHAB total general behaviour score has significant positive correlations with both anergia and the BPRS total score. These results show a strong relationship between social and behavioural functioning and psychiatric state at 12 months post-discharge.

Table 4.5
REHAB scores and BPRS Anergia Factor, BPRS total score;
Spearman correlation coefficients at 12 months post-discharge
(N = 29)

REHAB	Anergia	Total Score
Social Activity	.44**	.43**
Speech Skills	.47**	.22
Disturbed Speech	– .04	.27
Self Care	.24	.49**
Community Skills	.33*	.33*
Total General Behaviour Score	.37**	.48**

Significance * $p < 0.05$, ** $p < 0.01$

A pattern of considerable change in social and behavioural functioning is evident in the first twelve months of community living which indicates the impact of new environments and care practices on clients who have spent many years in hospital. The fact that the main improvements took place so soon after resettlement suggests that many clients had a potential to function at a higher level which had previously not been realised.

Outcomes in Community Care Scheme I and Community Care Scheme II

Community Care Scheme I and Community Care Scheme II account for 22 of the 29 subjects (75.86%) assessed at 12 months post-discharge. The care practices, care environments, and outcomes for these two groups are therefore particularly important for an understanding of the factors affecting those resettled in the early stages of their adjustment to the community. Analysis of the results for these two schemes is rendered more interesting because of their different environments and care practices which are focused on two distinct resident groups - 'old long-stay' and 'new long-stay' patients in hospital. Given the different baseline characteristics of the two groups in age, total time hospitalised, levels of psychiatric symptomatology and dependency levels one would anticipate different outcomes. The philosophy of care of each of the two community schemes had elements of similarity - a belief in the value of community involvement, respect for the privacy and rights of the individual and the offering of environments which were mainly domestic in character. It is equally clear that there were sharp distinctions between the two schemes in the approach to care practices. Scheme I pursued an objective of freedom, independence, choice and responsibility for the individual. Scheme II placed emphasis on involvement in domestic routines, responsibility for household chores, the creation of personalised domestic environments, care worker initiation of shopping and leisure activities and a 'family' atmosphere in each of the five houses making up the scheme. Data collected at hospital baseline and twelve months post-discharge have therefore been analysed and compared for each of the two schemes. The results of the psychiatric assessments are considered first. Analysis has been conducted to demonstrate the between subjects effects of placement by repeated assessments. Thus, the analysis was undertaken to show any effect of the community location on clients at the 12 months post-discharge assessment when compared with the data for the same groups while resident in hospital. This analysis takes account of the baseline scores for each of the two groups resettled to Scheme I and Scheme II and determines whether a significant difference arises as the result of placement in the community.

Mental state

Inspection of the BPRS total score (Table 4.6) shows that there are no significant differences between baseline assessment and 12 months post-discharge within each of the two schemes, although there is an initial significant difference between the schemes which persists over the period of the assessments. It has been noted earlier that active psychiatric symptomatology shows greater prevalence in Scheme I. There is some decrease for Scheme I - total score 20.5 (SD 13.54) to 16.71 (SD 17.24) while an increase in symptomatology occurs in Scheme II - 5.0 (SD 6.0) to 8.07 (SD 7.83).

Table 4.6
Brief Psychiatric Rating Scale (BPRS) Scheme I and Scheme II hospital baseline and 12 months post-discharge (N=22)

	Hospital Baseline		12 months Post-discharge		Between Subjects Effects Placement by Repeat (significance for T2 using unique sum of squares)
Anxiety-Depression	M	(SD)	M	(SD)	F Ratio
Scheme I	1.39	(1.4)	1.35	(1.6)	3.37
Scheme II	0.09	(0.24)	0.46	(0.44)	
Anergia					
Scheme I	0.57	(0.63)	0.05	(0.12)	0.78
Scheme II	0.53	(1.15)	0.41	(0.67)	
Thought Disturbance					
Scheme I	2.12	(1.77)	1.58	(1.87)	1.57
Scheme II	0.43	(0.54)	0.5	(1.15)	
Activation					
Scheme I	0.82	(0.88)	0.92	(0.78)	0.00
Scheme II	0.61	(0.74)	0.71	(0.66)	
Hostility - Suspiciousness					
Scheme I	1.02	(1.07)	0.97	(1.37)	2.16
Scheme II	0.95	(0.27)	0.61	(0.83)	
BPRS Total Score					
Scheme I	20.5	(13.54)	16.71	(17.24)	3.24
Scheme II	5.0	(6.0)	8.07	(7.83)	
No significant results					

However, in terms of overall levels of symptomatology Scheme I still shows significantly higher levels of active symptoms at the 12 months post-discharge assessment (F=6.90, P<.05). The differences between the two schemes are associated with the mean age of residents, higher levels of psychiatric symptomatology being prevalent in the younger group. No significant difference over time emerges in an analysis of placement by repeat assessment, which indicates that there has not been an interaction between factors associated with the community care settings, such as care management or care environment, and the outcomes in terms of psychiatric symptomatology. Turning to the factor scores, there are significant differences in anxiety levels between the schemes which persist over time. Scheme I residents continue to show higher anxiety levels (F=6.99, P<.05) and greater levels of thought disturbance (F=6.33, P<.05) in comparison to the Scheme II group. An inspection of individual BPRS items shows that residents in Scheme II have lower levels of anxiety (F=8.35, P<.01), depression (F=7.36, P<.01), guilt (F=4.39, P<.05), unusual thought content (F=5.57, P<.05), grandiosity (F= 7.83, P<.01) and hallucinations (F=5.64, P<.05) compared to Scheme I residents. No significant differences between the two groups of clients emerged from the SANS-AF ratings at 12 months post-discharge (Table 4.7) in the analysis of placement by repeat assessment.

Table 4.7
Scale for the Assessment of Negative Symptoms (SANS-AF)
Scheme I and Scheme II
hospital baseline and 12 months post-discharge (N=22)

		Hospital Baseline	12 months Post-discharge	Placement by Repeat (Significance for T2 using unique sum of squares)
		M (SD)	M (SD)	F Ratio
Facial Expressiveness	Scheme I	0.83(0.98)	0.33 (0.82)	0.03
	Scheme II	1.08(1.16)	0.46 (0.97)	
Spontaneous Movement	Scheme I	0.16(0.41)	0.54 (1.30)	0.09
	Scheme II	0.33(0.82)	0.54 (1.13)	
Expressive Gestures	Scheme I	0.5 (0.83)	0.33 (0.82)	0.13
	Scheme II	0.62(1.56)	0.69 (1.49)	
Eye Contact	Scheme I	0.5 (0.84)	0.5 (0.84)	0.09
	Scheme II	0.58(1.40)	0.75 (1.14)	
Affective Responsivity	Scheme I	0.33(0.82)	0.33 (0.82)	0.09
	Scheme II	0.54(1.39)	0.39 (0.96)	
Vocal Inflexion	Scheme I	0.83(0.98)	0.5 (0.84)	0.36
	Scheme II	0.53(1.39)	0.54 (1.23)	

No significant results

Turning to the KRS, Scheme II residents show lower levels of depression (F=6.16, P<.05), anxiety (F=6.82, P<.01), delusions (F=4.77, P<.05) and hallucinations (F=5.04, P<.05) than Scheme I residents (Table 4.8). These initial differences between the two groups persisted at the 12 months post discharge assessment and there were no significant differences in placement by repeat assessment.

To summarise, the initial differences in psychiatric symptomatology between these two groups at hospital baseline persist at the 12 months post-discharge assessment. This demonstrates that in the first 12 months the changed care environments and care practices have had little impact on levels of active psychiatric symptomatology and that significant between scheme differences over time have not emerged in either of the two care schemes.

Table 4.8

Krawiecka Rating Scale (KRS) Scheme I and Scheme II
hospital baseline and 12 months post-discharge (N=22)

	Hospital Baseline		12 months Post-discharge		Placement by Repeat (Significance for T2 using unique sum of squares)
Depression	M	(SD)	M	(SD)	F Ratio
Scheme I	0.85	(1.49)	0.85	(1.21)	0.9
Scheme II	0.11	(0.30)	0.00	(0.00)	
Anxiety					
Scheme I	1.57	(0.83)	1.28	(1.25)	2.18
Scheme II	0.34	(0.55)	0.76	(0.92)	
Delusion					
Scheme I	2.57	(1.90)	1.57	(1.98)	3.98
Scheme II	0.42	(1.08)	0.85	(1.70)	
Hallucination					
Scheme I	1.71	(2.13)	1.51	(1.98)	0.15
Scheme II	0.23	(0.83)	0.30	(1.10)	
Incoherence					
Scheme I	1.00	(1.15)	0.14	(0.37)	2.34
Scheme II	0.60	(1.07)	0.92	(1.54)	
Poverty Speech					
Scheme I	0.71	(0.18)	0.00	(0.00)	0.33
Scheme II	0.80	(1.37)	0.93	(1.03)	
Flattened Affect					
Scheme I	0.35	(0.37)	0.35	(0.62)	0.03
Scheme II	0.53	(0.99)	0.46	(0.91)	
Psycho-motor retardation					
Scheme I	0.28	(0.39)	0.00	(0.00)	1.88
Scheme II	0.26	(0.70)	0.30	(0.59)	

No significant results

Social and behavioural functioning

The analysis of the REHAB results for Scheme I and Scheme II reveals a very different situation from the psychiatric assessments. Inspection of the total general behaviour score shows that significant changes have taken place in the two schemes by twelve months post-discharge. In Scheme I the total general behavioural score has deteriorated from 30.64 (SD 20.21) to 42.07 (SD 21.15), while in Scheme II the score has improved from 61.92 (SD 24.82) to 44.34 (SD 24.12) (F=13.71, P<.01) (Table 4.9). The result indicates a statistically significant interaction between placement and the outcome measured by the REHAB total general behaviour score. Analysis measuring the simple separate main effect of change in each scheme shows that the result is significant for Scheme II (F=11.91, P<.002) but not for Scheme I (F=2.97, p<.095). We may therefore conclude that it is the change in the score for Scheme II which is predominant in determining the significant placement by repeat assessment result. The deterioration in the result for Scheme I is not statistically significant. In fact, a preliminary inspection of results for the following assessment point (2 years post-hospital discharge) shows that the deterioration at twelve months post-discharge was a temporary phenomenon, the score at two years post-discharge being 29.06, which is marginally better than hospital baseline.

Table 4.9
Hall & Baker REHAB Scheme I and Scheme II
hospital baseline and 12 months post-discharge (N=22)

REHAB	Hospital Baseline		12 months Post-discharge		Placement by Repeat (Significance for T2 using unique sum of squares)
Social Activity	M	(SD)	M	(SD)	F Ratio
Scheme I	12.85	(8.45)	20.14	(10.07)	11.95**
Scheme II	25.34	(13.8)	15.35	(11.58)	
Speech Skills					
Scheme I	2.64	(3.5)	4.07	(2.47)	6.35**
Scheme II	7.03	(4.7)	3.57	(4.16)	
Disturbed Speech					
Scheme I	3.92	(3.66)	2.00	(1.08)	.00
Scheme II	4.57	(3:88)	3.96	(2.74)	
Self Care					
Scheme I	6.5	(7.09)	9.64	(8.53)	3.64
Scheme II	16.07	(10.39)	12.92	(7.62)	
Community Skills					
Scheme I	5.5	(4.68)	6.5	(3.88)	11.32**
Scheme II	11.32	(5.87)	7.07	(5.1)	
Total General Behaviour Score					
Scheme I	30.64	(20.21)	42.07	(22.15)	
Scheme II	61.92	(24.82)	44.34	(24.12)	13.71**

Significance ** P <0.01

Examination of the REHAB Factor Scores shows that significant change by time and placement has occurred in three of the five Factors. Social activity has decreased for residents in Scheme I but has increased for those in Scheme II ($F=11.95$, $p<.01$), speech skills have deteriorated in Scheme I, but improved in Scheme II ($F=6.35$, $P<.01$) and community skills have deteriorated in Scheme I but improved in Scheme II ($F=11.32$, $P< .01$). These changes in the factor scores largely account for the change in the total general behaviour score. They indicate that the nature of the change taking place is concerned with social interaction and community involvement. It should be noted that the significant changes over time by placement are mainly accounted for improvements in Scheme II residents. These changes had largely taken place by the time of the six weeks post-discharge assessment (Figure 4.3). These results mark significant changes related to placement from hospital baseline to twelve months post discharge.

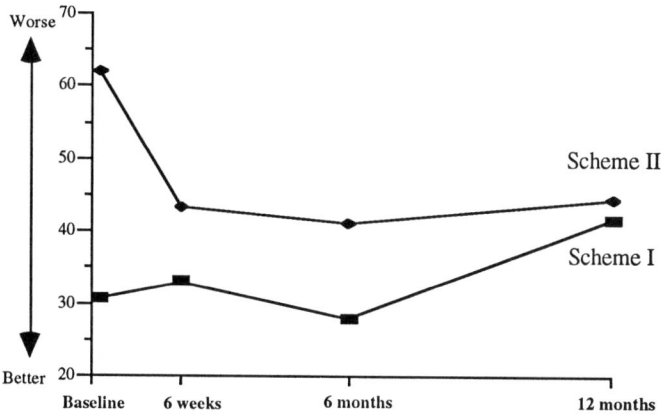

Clinical Judgements
Potential for discharge - total general behaviour score < 40
moderate handicap   - total general behaviour score 41 - 60
severe handicap   - total general behaviour score > - 61

Figure 4.3
Hall & Baker REHAB
Mean total general behaviour scores
Hospital baseline, 6 weeks, 6 months and 12 months post-discharge

Results for those remaining in hospital

An assessment of those remaining in hospital at a point corresponding to the 12 months post-discharge assessment for those returned to the community revealed some interesting comparisons. With regard to psychiatric state, the BPRS Total Score shows some deterioration over baseline for those remaining in hospital, although this is not a statistically significant result (Table 4.10). It has previously been noted that there was a slight improvement in the BPRS Total Score for those resettled to the community. The fact that neither of these results is significant suggests that mental state is remaining stable in both the hospital stayers and the community group. Such stability over time is probably attributable to the maintenance of medication in both groups.

Turning to the results of the SANS -AF (Table 4.11) it will be noted that while there has been an improvement in all items for those living in the community, comparing the twelve months post-discharge assessment with hospital baseline, there has been a deterioration for the hospital stayers on all items except vocal inflection.

Table 4.10
Brief Psychiatric Rating Scale (BPRS) hospital stayers (N=17) and Community Care Schemes I and II (N=22) hospital baseline and 12 months post-discharge

	Hospital Baseline	12-Months Post-Discharge	F-Ratio
Hospital	10.86 (6.66)	13.13 (9.37)	1.17
Community Schemes I & II	12.64 (12.79)	11.89 (9.98)	0.23

No significant results

In consequence, while there was no statistically significant difference between the two groups at baseline a significant difference has developed in the overall result at the twelve months post-discharge assessment point (F=6.88, p<.01).

Table 4.11
Scale for the Assessment of Negative Symptoms (SANS-AF) hospital stayers (N=17) and Community Care Schemes I and II (N=22) hospital baseline and 12 months post-discharge

		Hospital Baseline	12-Months Post-Discharge
Facial Expressiveness	Hospital	0.85 (1.46)	1.14 (1.24)
	Community Schemes I & II	0.83 (1.09)	0.17 (0.40)
Spontaneous Movement	Hospital	0.28 (0.82)	0.50 (0.83)
	Community Schemes I & II	0.45 (0.81)	0.33 (0.18)
Expressive Gestures	Hospital	0.57 (1.01)	0.64 (1.00)
	Community Schemes I & II	0.58 (1.31)	0.13 (0.52)
Eye Contact	Hospital	0.71 (1.20)	0.92 (1.28)
	Community Schemes I & II	0.77 (1.40)	0.41 (1.11)
Affective Responsivety	Hospital	0.78 (1.47)	0.96 (1.32)
	Community Schemes I & II	0.51 (1.09)	0.13 (0.43)
Vocal Inflection	Hospital	0.64 (1.15)	0.35 (0.92)
	Community Schemes I & II	0.80 (1.10)	0.25 (0.74)
Significance ** p<0.01		F = 0.04	F = 6.88**

Inspection of the REHAB Deviant Behaviour Scores comparing those resettled in the community with those remaining in hospital shows that while there has been a slight improvement for those moving to the community and a slight deterioration for those remaining in hospital, there is no statistically significant effect of placement by repeated assessment (Table 4.12).

Analysis of the REHAB Total General Behaviour Score shows that there has been improvement for those remaining in hospital, although this is not statistically significant. There has been a greater improvement for those resettled from the hospital to Community Scheme II and this change is statistically significant as noted previously (F=11.91, p<.01) (Table 4.13).

It is possible that the non-significant improvement in the result for those remaining in hospital is attributable to the effect of rehabilitation programmes, which are seeking to develop self-care skills and independence for patients prior to resettlement.

Table 4.12
Hall & Baker REHAB deviant behaviour scores
for hospital stayers (N=17) and Community Care Schemes I & II
hospital baseline and 12 months post-discharge

		Hospital Baseline	12-Months Post-Discharge	F-Ratio
Hospital	N=17	1.51 (1.29)	1.71 (1.26)	1.50
Community Schemes I & II	N=22	1.34 (1.19)	1.20 (1.14)	
No significant results				

Overall, the comparison of outcomes for those remaining in hospital with those now in the community shows that the improvements evident in the community group have not been matched by those in the hospital.

Table 4.13
Hall & Baker REHAB
total general behaviour scores for hospital stayers (N=17)
and Community Care Schemes I & II
hospital baseline and 12 months post-discharge

		Hospital Baseline	12-Months Post-Discharge	F-Ratio
Hospital	N = 17	64.00 (24.94)	53.84 (25.90)	3.97
Scheme I	N = 8	30.64 (20.21)	42.07 (22.15)	2.97
Scheme II	N = 14	61.92 (24.82)	44.34 (24.12)	11.91 **
Significance ** p<0.01				

Discussion

The results from the psychiatric assessments, comparing hospital baseline and 12 months post-discharge suggest that resettlement has not resulted in a deterioration in psychiatric symptomatology in the resettlement group as a whole. The absence of significant change in the BPRS total score supports this overall conclusion. Within this overview there have been a number of significant changes in item scores and factor scores. The decrease in blunted affect, emotional withdrawal and reduction in the anergia factor score (BPRS), together with increased facial expressiveness and spontaneous movements (SANS-AF) correlate with an increase in levels of stimulation and engagement in social interaction for members of the resettlement group. The significant reduction in long term depression (KRS) may also be attributable to a common factor associated with higher levels of stimulation in community settings. The increase in the BPRS hostility-suspiciousness score is more difficult to interpret, although it may be viewed as a response to the increased demands and uncertainties encountered in the move to new situations and care practices, in which there are increased levels of uncertainty, greater responsibility for decision-making and new social situations which require adjustment by individuals. These results are similar to those identified by the TAPS project (Anderson, et al., 1993) after twelve months community residence. They noted some minor variations in psychiatric symptomatology but found that overall levels of symptomatology were stable. "The fact is that the one year data suggests that the psychiatric state of these long-stay patients was stable whether they left hospital or remained there" (p53). The changes which have occurred in social and behavioural functioning are more pronounced, with a significant improvement in the total general behaviour score (REHAB) at 12 months post-discharge. The changes observed in the psychiatric ratings and the behavioural assessments should not be viewed in isolation, but should be seen as interrelated outcome variables, which reflect changed environments and care practices. Medical supervision in the community provided continuity in medication and the stabilisation of symptoms.

The analysis of data for the two groups resettled to Care Scheme I and Care Scheme II provides greater insight into the processes by which changes have occurred in the move to community care. Significant differences existed between the two groups at baseline assessment in terms of psychiatric symptomatology (BPRS total score) and social functioning (REHAB total general behaviour score). The group which has been characterised as 'old long-stay' patients had significantly lower levels of active psychiatric symptomatology than the 'new long-stay' group. The initial differences in psychiatric symptomatology have persisted and no significant variance over time by placement has been identified. Similar findings have been noted for the KRS and SANS-AF results. The outcomes with regard to social and behavioural functioning provide real evidence of change over time and show clear improvement in Scheme II. The explanation of these significant changes must lie in an interaction between clients' characteristics and the different care processes espoused by the two schemes.

It has already been noted that the approach to care in Scheme I emphasised independence and freedom. The antipathy to institutionalisation and the collective treatment of individuals was represented by a determination to eschew hospital practices. It was expressed in a reluctance to adopt directive practices (such as organising group outings). The degree to which this approach to care practices has been implemented is reflected in the extremely low score for restrictive practices observed in the result for the Hospital-Hospices Practices Profile. In Scheme II there has been a reduction in the extent to which care practices are restrictive, but not to the extent observed in Scheme I. Behavioural expectations are still established for individuals, group activities are organised, staff frequently take residents out to shops and cafés. This scheme promotes a degree of structure which is intended to support its 'old long-stay' clients in the transition to a greater degree of self determination in the community. In Scheme I it is anticipated that the 'new long-stay' residents may wish to move to more independent living, for example a house or flat linked to the Scheme. In Scheme II residents are expected to be cared for in the same setting for life. This perhaps explains the results of different care philosophies which are evident in the data presented in this chapter. In both community schemes medical supervison by consultants and community psychiatric nurses has ensured continuity of medical care. Community staff have continued to ensure compliance with medication. It is not surprising, therefore, that changes in psychiatric symptomatology have been limited, and largely confined to aspects which are more amenable to influence by increased levels of stimulation. In this respect the move to community care has ensured continuity, while expanding the opportunity for social participation and social support considerably. Scheme I and Scheme II have provided for two essentially different client groups. Nonetheless, the behavioural outcomes do suggest that care practices which place initial maximum importance on independence may not be the most effective way of developing renewed responsibility for, and control of, one's life for individuals who have lived in a hospital environment which engendered a dependency culture. It should also be born in mind that it is often suggested that schizophrenia is characterised by a lack of motivation and initiative which could contribute to the development of a dependency culture. To combat this requires well resourced care schemes and high levels of staff motivation to promote the involvement of clients in social activities. The TAPS study found that clients had developed wider social networks after twelve months in the community. It remains to be seen whether a similar development will occur for clients in the present study. It is clear, however, that the opportunity framework for such a development exists to a greater extent in the community than in the hospital. The REHAB factor scores, which are implicated in the result of the total general behaviour score - social activity, speech skills, and community skills – are the most directly affected by care practices. It is particularly interesting to note that all the residents of Scheme II came from the one hospital ward which had the most deprived conditions - the lowest staff: client ratio, the least occupational therapy inputs, the least qualified staff and the lowest costs of care. The observation study undertaken in this ward prior to resettlement indicated the paucity of social stimulation and a general lack of activity. This most deprived group of hospital patients was moved into the best resourced community care setting with the highest staff: client ratio, the most domestic environment and most costly care provision. It might be tempting to conclude that the greater the cost the better the result. This could be misleading. These results should rather be interpreted as the realisation of a potential which was not being tapped while individuals remained in the most stagnant ward environment investigated. The patients who were to move to Scheme I were already functioning at a higher level in hospital. A levelling up in social and behavioural functioning has occurred for those resident in Scheme II, which results in a similar score for both groups at 12 months post-discharge. It should also be noted that these results can not be regarded as the final outcome for either group. Both may be expected to experience a more protracted period of adjustment to life out of hospital in view of their lengthy experience of hospitalisation. Indeed, the very immediacy of the improvement in the 'old long-stay' group suggests that a deprived situation had been rectified. More fundamental changes in both groups are likely to take place over a longer period of time.

In both groups there is a preference for their new community lives over the hospital environment. This should be regarded as a positive indication of the benefits which both groups have experienced as a result of changes in policy which have led to the resettlement of 'old long-stay' patients who have spent most of their lives in hospital and 'new long-stay' patients who would have shared their experience had not policy changed.

Attention has been focused on the 75% of respondents who had been resettled in the two community care schemes, because it is possible to trace clearly the link between care environments, care practices and outcomes in these schemes. Such a detailed examination has not been possible for those resettled to private care homes, social services homes for the elderly, and those who have moved to live with family. The number of these individuals is small (8) and their relocation in various settings makes it impossible to establish a clear connection between care practices and outcomes. As a group, the psychiatric and behavioural outcomes do not vary significantly from the results established for the total resettlement group. Comment should however be made on the two people relocated to independent living. Both were 'new long-stay' patients and both have experienced subsequent hospital readmissions. If the focus of care management in the community is to be the integrated delivery of services (Ford et al., 1993) it should also be born in mind that support must be sufficient to sustain community tenure for vulnerable individuals. The issue of social support as well as achieving integrated services for those who move to live in less sheltered accommodation merits further investigation.

Conclusion

The discussion of care practices and care environments has provided a key to understanding outcomes of care. The results of this study suggest that care practices and environments can be related to the outcomes for client groups. In this study care practices and the care environment in hospital have been shown to be related to the lower levels of social and behavioural functioning identified in one group of 'old long-stay' clients. Improved quality of care has resulted in significantly improved levels of functioning for a group which appeared not to be realising its full potential. These 'old long-stay' patients have experienced an improved level of social and behavioural functioning as a result of the move to a well resourced community care scheme. The increased staff: client ratio can be identified as one factor in the improved quality of care experienced by this group. Perhaps more important are the changes in care environment - from an isolated location to normal housing areas which are close to community facilities. Equally important is the philosophy of care and new care management practices, which emphasise participation and integration. The positive motivation of staff to their care roles is essential if the objectives of care schemes are to be achieved.

The results for 'new long-stay' hospital patients show higher initial levels of social and behavioural functioning in rather more stimulating ward environments, with care practices which were more actively directed to rehabilitation. The improvements noted in 'old long-stay' patients are not evident in this group, which was relocated to Scheme I, with less directive care practices. Because of the different initial characteristics of the two groups it is not be possible to conclude that one type of care practice is superior to the other in terms of social and behavioural functioning outcomes. However, the results do suggest that it may well be worth testing more actively interventionist care practices with 'new long-stay' clients as well as the 'old long-stay' groups.

Despite this limitation, when the results of the North Wales Study are examined it may be concluded that service users have gained in the move from hospital to local care settings. Their psychiatric state has tended to remain stable in the community and there have been some significant improvements in level of engagement, associated with less restrictive care regimes, which have placed care planning for the individual client at the centre of care management.

Clients themselves have reported finding considerable improvement over the hospital environment in freedom and independence and have evaluated the new care settings and care practices positively (see chapter 6). Care in the community has produced positive gains and few significant losses for those who have moved to live in well resourced care schemes which offer a combination of professional and social support. The difficulties faced by those relocated to isolated, independent living have been illustrated by the two subjects placed in such situations, who have experienced rehospitalisation. It can be concluded that care in the community is effective when care environments and care practices provide appropriate levels of support in adequately resourced schemes. Such provision is not a cheap alternative (see chapter 7), but need not be any more expensive than hospital care. The transformation in diminished lives of those 'old long-stay' patients in this study, who had spent most of their lives in hospital, provides a strong impetus for change. The study of outcomes for clients already resettled and those yet to be resettled is continuing. When it is completed it will be possible to draw conclusions concerning the effects of resettlement for all those in the research cohort.

References

Anderson, J., Dayson, D., Wills, W., Gooch, C., Margolius, O., O'Driscoll, C., Leff, J. 'The TAPS Project: Clinical and social outcomes of long-stay psychiatric patients after one year in the community' in J. Leff, (ed), 1993 'The TAPS Project: Evaluating Community Placement of Long-Stay Psychiatric Patients', *British Journal of Psychiatry*. Vol 162, Supplement 19.

Baker, R., Hall, J.N. (1983), *Users' Manual for Rehabiliation Evaluation of Hall and Baker*. Vine Publishing Ltd. Aberdeen.

Crosby, C., Barry, M.M., Carter, M.F., Lowe, C.F. (1993), 'Psychiatric Rehabilitation and Community Care: Resettlement from a North Wales Hospital', *Heath and Social Care in the Community*. 1, pp355-363.

Clwyd Health Authority (1991), *Clwyd Plan for Mental Illness Services*. Clwyd Health Authority, Mold.

Ford, R., Repper, J., Cooke, A., Norton, P., Beadsmoore, A., Clark, C. (1993), 'Implementing Case Management: Research report on the process of developing case management services for people with a long-term mental illness'. R.D.P. London.

Welsh Office (1989) *Mental Illness Services: A Strategy for Wales*. Welsh Office, Cardiff.

5 Social networks and lives of people with long-term mental health problems

Rachel Forrester-Jones and Gordon Grant

Summary

Relying on an applied social network analysis and case study material, this chapter describes patterns of social relationships as individuals begin to construct new lives in the community following lengthy periods of hospitalisation. The findings indicate how experiences can be mediated by different care practices in alternative housing schemes. Also indicated are tensions between maintaining the solidarity of existing long-term relationships between individuals and their associates, and the creation of opportunities to fashion new relationships in the community. The chapter ends with some reflections on policy and practice.

Background

With the movement of significant numbers of people from long-stay psychiatric hospitals to the community as hospitals are de-commissioned, interesting opportunities are presented to examine how individuals adapt to a new life. The recent care in the community demonstration projects have illustrated the organisational, economic and personal benefits that can be associated with living in the community as opposed to long-stay hospital (Knapp et. al., 1992) and this experience has been greatly influential in shaping the provisions of the NHS and Community Care Act 1990. The evaluation of the care in the community demonstration projects has generated an enormous amount of policy relevant data but without much emphasis on the first hand experiences and social situation of service users. In the present case, the closure of the North Wales Hospital (NWH), created the prospect of a small-scale but intensive study concerned with the social life of individuals shortly after their relocation to community-based housing schemes.

The prevailing policy emphasis on the mixed economy of welfare by many countries of the developed world has created renewed interest in the notion of social networks and how support can be elicited from them to sustain people who may be disadvantaged. Popular views have developed that such support, especially from families, can under normal circumstances be expected to be relatively enduring. However, studies show that informal support can be a highly variable commodity in terms of its availability, scope, stability and adaptability (Grant and Wenger, 1993) and there are major questions to be asked about whether, and under what circumstances, such support can be reinforced by formal agencies (D'Abbs, 1982; Gottlieb, 1981; Yoder et al., 1985; Whittaker and Garbarino, 1983).

The variety of functions that informal support serves for individuals has generated different theoretical approaches to the study of social support. It has been argued for example that there are at least three discernible theoretical approaches: human ecology theory, social support and social network theory, and help-seeking and help-giving theory (Dunst et al., 1989). Human ecology theory appears to derive from the early work of Bronfenbrenner (1979) and has principally been focused on understanding the direct and indirect impact on human development of a wide variety of ecologically conceived systems and units such as families, neighbourhoods, and formal organisations. Social support and social network theory is based on understanding relationships between different social units and how these promote or impede the flow and exchange of social support and other resources (Gottlieb, 1981). Social support is viewed multi-dimensionally and is usually construed as including physical or practical assistance (Pattison, 1977), information (Kahn and Antonucci, 1980), emotional support (House, 1981), attitude transmission (Barrera and Ainlay, 1983), and gatekeeping to other resources. Social networks may be viewed as the opportunity framework or structure through which social support is provided. Literature within the social support and social network field has arguably had the greatest impact on policy thinking in developed countries, and it has had a major influence in shaping this particular study. Help-seeking and help-giving theory appears to have its roots in American community psychology and is based mostly on analysis of the interdependencies between help seekers and givers (Fisher, Nadler and DePaulo, 1983; Gourash, 1978).

Social support network characteristics have been shown to be related to the adjustment of individuals in a variety of contexts. For example, the social and clinical functioning of people with schizophrenia appears to be linked to the structural and interpersonal characteristics of the networks of closest associates (Taylor, Huxley and Johnson, 1984). Support networks, in varying degrees, also insulate people from depression (Brown and Harris, 1978) as well as from anxiety (Henderson et al., 1980) and minor affective disorders (Brugha et al., 1982).

Within the prevailing context of deinstitutionalisation, studies have shown that successful discharge is related to employment and relationship to those to whom the person returns (Brown et al., 1958). More recent studies such as those of TAPS (Team for the Assessment of Psychiatric Services, 1993) indicate that social networks are potentially protective against stress and repeated breakdown of those discharged from hospital (Dunn et al., 1990). Indeed, O'Driscoll and Leff (1993) in their study of long-stay patients discharged from two hospitals to an inner-London Health District found that 'one of the main anxieties being expressed both by and on behalf of patients leaving a mental hospital is the possible disruption to their social networks'. Furthermore, Dunn et. al. (1990) argue that social networks mediate successful reintegration into the community. Thornicroft and Breakey (1991) investigated social networks of 97 long-term mentally ill patients living in inner-city Baltimore who were in contact with the COSTAR programme - a mobile treatment and case management service for the long-term mentally ill. They found that supportive and intimate personal relationships can guard against social isolation and are associated with better outcome such as cognitive function. Substantiating this, Dayson (1992) argues that good social relationships are associated with, even if not necessarily causes of, good outcomes in chronic schizophrenia. Similarly, Baker et al., (1977) found that those returning into the community to larger and more socially diverse networks adjusted better socially and occupationally than others with smaller more closed networks.

Within related fields of study, kinship networks reflecting different orientations to involvement with adults with a learning disability have been reported to be related to levels of achievement in terms of independent living and employment (Winik, Zetlin and Kaufman, 1985). Amongst children, including those with special needs, network dynamics have been shown to be related to child, parent and family functioning (Dunst and Trivette, 1988; Zarling, Hirsch and Landry, 1988), whilst amongst families with young children in general, support network type have been linked to patterns of child abuse and neglect (Crittenden, 1985). Indeed, reviews indicate that the incidence of suicides, homicides, car accidents, alcoholism, and proneness to accidents can all be related to the presence or absence of support networks (D'Abbs 1982; Pilisuk and Froland, 1978).

Network size and membership are key dimensions of support network structures. Size, or the number of network members identified, appears to be one of the most commonly assessed structural parameters of networks (Sokolovsky et. al., 1978; Huxley, 1984; Walker et. al., 1975). It is thought that there is a relationship between the number of contacts and psychopathology, with smaller networks being in evidence for individuals with schizophrenia (Pattison et. al., 1975; Thornicroft and Breakey 1991), than for general population samples. In terms of membership, the literature on informal support networks has shown a relationship between membership category and function within social networks. For example, members linked through kinship appear to be the main providers of instrumental, emotional and economic support for aged and disabled relatives over time whilst friends and neighbours play more subsidiary but complementary roles (Wenger 1984, Grant and Wenger 1993). These studies also suggest that, with changes in support network membership, substitutability of support between categories of members can occur. Network size and membership therefore provide a first indication of the potential human support available to individuals.

Studies have tended to concentrate on the structural properties of networks like size, density, membership and linkages, perhaps because these are the most amenable for study. Latterly there has been more interest in the function or content of relationships embedded within social networks and it is this which has been described as the most important item of information about networks as it indicates something of the goods and services exchanged, the closeness or intimacy between members, the intensity of their interactions and the exchange of information involved (Bulmer, 1987).

More recently it has been argued that it is much less clear what it is about social relationships that affects health and how these effects occur. House, Umberson and Landis (1988) contend that three aspects of social relationships - their existence and quantity, their formal structure, and their functional content - must be conceptually and empirically distinguished. These were termed social integration, social networks and relational content respectively. The concept of social support is one type of relational content, the others being suggested as (i) relational demands and conflicts and (ii) social regulation or control. Social integration and networks can be seen as representing structures of social relationships that may affect health while social support, relational demands and regulation are social processes through which these structures may have their effects.

Whilst social network studies provide vital clues about health and behaviour, Rook (1992) provides a timely reminder that social support provided by social network members may also be construed negatively by recipients either because the provided support is not needed, or more or less than what is needed, or support provided engenders a false sense of self-efficacy. Studies aimed at elucidating whether and how community care works for individuals need therefore to take into account the nature of the opportunity structure of support as well as the characteristics of the support itself and how this is construed.

Applying a social support and social network approach to the field of community mental health

The basic idea of the study was twofold. Firstly, with the resettlement of long-stay patients from the NWH to community settings with opportunities to develop new social networks, it was a chance to re-examine whether the assumed relative poverty of the networks of people with long-term psychiatric conditions necessarily holds. It was decided to test this out by assessing the structural properties of the networks of the individuals concerned. However, it was considered that this would be a rather sterile exercise without attempting to explore the processes through which these structures have their effects. Accordingly, the second dimension to the study was to be concerned with how individuals came to attribute meanings to the relationships that had developed between themselves and other people. The methodological approach was one which relied heavily on triangulation of methods and pluralistic evaluation (Smith and Cantley, 1985). More is said of this below.

The study context

The social network study ran in parallel to a comparative evaluation of institutional and community mental health services conducted by the Health Services Research Unit (HSRU) at the University of Wales, Bangor. This involved a large-scale longitudinal study of individuals' psychiatric state, behaviour and quality of life the results of which are presented in this book. In order to maintain the anonymity of the clients involved in this study, all individual names have been changed.

The study was based on community mental health housing projects based in two rural communities. The first, Scheme I, was situated within a North Wales town, close to the North Wales Hospital, to which ten of the subject group were relocated.

Table 5.1
Details of study sample

		Scheme I	Scheme II	Total
Sample number		10	15	25
Gender:	men	8	14	22
	women	2	1	3
Age range		37-65	58-79	37-79
Mean age		49	68	61
Age first hospitalised		18-38	12-42	12-42
No. of hospitalisations		1-23	1-7	1-23
Ave. yrs. hospitalised		15	30	26
Diagnosis:				
Schizophrenia				83%

Scheme II was situated within another North Wales market town, some eight miles from the North Wales Hospital. Fifteen subjects were resettled here. The study sample is a sub-sample of the research cohort described in chapter 2.

Summary details of the study sample are given in Table 5.1. None of the residents were in full-time employment but were in receipt of social security benefits i.e. income support and invalidity benefit. No-one had been in paid employment since hospitalisation. Prior to hospitalisation, eleven residents had worked as labourers, three as semi-skilled labourers, four as skilled manual workers, and one as a skilled non-manual worker. Using the Standard Occupational Classification Scale (HMSO 1991), two individuals were in social class I and II, five in III and fourteen in IV and V. Four individuals had never worked but three of these were in higher education at the time of their hospitalisation. Findings from the linked resettlement study showed that psychiatric symptomatology of individuals had changed little since hospital discharge but there had been some significant improvements in social and behavioural functioning (see chapter 4) and residents reported that they were satisfied with their life in the community (see chapter 6).

Method

A pilot study was carried out in the NWH where semi-structured, unstructured interviews and observations were carried out. This proved to be an invaluable introduction to the study participants. It was also instructive to gain background knowledge of the environment which had been home to many of the residents for on average 26 years. The pilot study revealed that either individuals can have difficulty recalling the names of people with whom they have contact or that they do not wish to identify their contacts. Difficulties in communication have been reported before in the psychiatric literature (Wallace 1984). In practical terms this meant that a method needed to be found for weighing the reliability of data obtained from the participants in this study. The study was also concerned with trying to understand the meaning and significance of support to individuals, something best understood through participant observation.

These considerations led to a fusion of quantitative and qualitative research methods. Support network structure was mapped initially through the use of an interview schedule based on the Social Network Schedule (SNS) (Dunn et al., 1990). The SNS was developed and used by the Team for the Assessment of Psychiatric Services (TAPS) with the remit of studying and evaluating the closure process of two London psychiatric hospitals. The SNS consisted of a name eliciting procedure using a time budget of the previous month to illuminate any usual social contacts identifiable by name or role. Further questions concerned the relative quality of contacts. The schedule was subsequently adapted for use with the participants in this study. Yearly was chosen as the boundary line for frequency of contact as the pilot study had indicated that although some individuals' contacts were seen only periodically, they were in fact meaningful and important to them in a variety of respects. This time-scale meant that network membership cut across both hospital and community settings. The second part of the SNS which concentrated on the quality of contacts was also adapted. It was felt that the original questions concerned with quality of relationships were a crude measure of intimacy and inappropriate for formal interviewing. The schedule was therefore adapted to include questions which referred to helping behaviours. More detailed questioning referring to intimacy of network members was left to later unstructured interviewing. Further modifications included the use of a diagrammatical family tree to record kin members and the use of a network member summary sheet.

Experience with the Social Network Interview (adapted SNS) suggested that it was failing to identify the 'whole' picture of an individual's network. One reason for this was that residents were sensitive to questions about their contacts. In particular, two residents from Scheme I displayed quite strong feelings of paranoia when asked about the people they knew. Since the interview was structured and confidential, it was necessary for the interviewer to sit down on a one-to-one basis with the interviewee. Although every effort was made to ask the questions in a relaxed atmosphere, there was still the sense that it was an 'interview' and individuals who have had to answer questions from psychiatrists and clinicians for many years did not necessarily adapt easily to what was still construed by them as a rather formal if not diagnostic event. Semi-structured interviews were also carried out to give residents a further opportunity to talk about their social lives, especially their patterns of daily living and their contacts with and participation in the community. It was anticipated that these fuller discussions might lead to the identification of more people who play potentially significant roles in their lives. One of the authors (R.F-J.) also spent a significant period of time living in with the residents and joining in activities with them so as to ascertain how their support networks were constituted and, more importantly, how they were used.

The Social Network Interview was administered approximately six months post-hospital discharge. Network members that were named but had no contact with the participant were recorded but not summated. The SNI was based on the week prior to interview to find out what activities individuals were engaged in and to elicit the names of contacts. More structured questions were also asked about frequency of contact. Further questions regarding the function as well as the content of relationships were also asked. Although this generated a considerable amount of data about support network structure, only details of size and membership are reported here.

In this chapter we have placed network members in one of the following categories although more detailed categorisation is to be published subsequently: family, staff, community members, hospital contacts or social acquaintances. Community members were local people in shops, post offices, hairdressers, general practitioners and others who were encountered more often than not in their occupational roles. Hospital contacts were other individuals who still were or had been resident in the psychiatric hospital. Staff included those who worked closely with

117

residents in their homes as well as social workers, community psychiatric nurses, psychiatrists and so forth, who would be expected to have more sporadic contact. Social acquaintances were those people who fitted into none of the aforementioned categories but who were nevertheless perceived by individuals as having some passing acquaintance sufficient for some sort of verbal exchange to have taken place on an occasional basis.

Results

Network Size

Social networks varied in size between 2 and 46 members, with a mean of 13.7 members. This is strikingly similar to findings reported by Thornicroft and Breakey (1991) who also used the SNS to interview 80 long-term psychiatric patients living in inner-city Baltimore in the USA. They found that the range for the number of group members was between 2 and 48 with a mean of 13.1. Moreover, Dunn et. al. (1990) found that for the ten patients in their hospital study, the network size ranged from 2 to 19 with a mode of 8 and a median of 8. In the present study the mode or most frequently occurring number of network members for this group was only six. However, as can be seen from Table 5.2 the size of network varies very considerably from individual to individual.

Network size varied appreciably between the two care schemes (Table 5.2). Those in Scheme I on average had larger networks, with six residents having networks consisting of 8 or more people whereas some residents in Scheme II had networks comprising as few as two people. To a degree this was predictable given that the two groups were of such different ages. As expected, family members of residents at Care Scheme II were either deceased or were not in contact.

Table 5.2.
Size and membership of individuals' social networks in two community care schemes

	Family		Staff		Community members		Hospital contacts		Social acquaintances		Total
	mean size	range	mean size	range	mean size	range	mean size	range	mean size	range	
Scheme I	2.8	0-6	5.3	0-11	0.2	0-2	7.7	1-12	0.6	0-2	16.5
Scheme II	1.2	0-4	4.5	1-17	1.6	0-11	4.5	1-17	0.2	0-4	12

This partly accounts for network size differences between the two groups. Furthermore, the two groups also consisted of individuals with different

118

communication skills, residents in Care Scheme II being initially more disabled than those in Care Scheme I. Residents in Scheme II were also more disabled for total general behaviour on the REHAB scale (Baker and Hall 1983) in comparison to residents in Scheme I, as reported in chapter 4.

At first sight, the data suggest that social networks are limited in size compared to those based on ordinary population samples which commonly report network sizes of over one hundred persons (for example, Sarason et. al., 1983). Such a stark difference highlights even more that individuals with mental health problems, particularly those hospitalised for lengthy periods, can have very impoverished networks in regard to size. However, since it is argued that different types of support come from different relationships (Weiss, 1969, 1974; Henderson, 1977) it could be argued that the potential for support is poor. This needs to be examined more closely in relation to network membership.

Membership

Network membership is an important parameter as it denotes the possible support functions that may be available to an individual. Although network membership details are given in Table 5.2 the distribution of network members of residents in the two housing schemes can be seen more easily in Figure 5.1. This shows for both schemes that the social relations of residents are comprised very largely of people connected to mental health services, that is staff, other residents or former associates from hospital. These groups account for 75% or more of residents' network members. Passing acquaintances with people whom residents might engage in conversation were not very evident for individuals in either scheme. The balance of network members was accounted for by family members. Individual differences in network membership are shown in Figure 5.2. Although exploration of individual differences is beyond the scope of this paper, more can be said about social network membership and distribution between the two care schemes.

Residents' networks were characterized by relatively few family members (ten had no kin as shown in Figure 5.2). Age and length of hospitalisation appear largely to account for this. Residents in Scheme I had slightly more family contacts than those in Scheme II. It was again probable that this was due to the fact that the average age of residents in Scheme I was nearly 20 years less then that of residents in Scheme II. In other words, the potential for contact with family was very much a function of life-cycle stage. However, for both groups the type of contact by family was the same. This comprised mostly of visits, telephone calls and, less frequently, letters.

Other residents, including former hospital associates, and staff were the most prominent members within individuals' networks. Individuals residing at Scheme I had more staff contacts than those at Scheme II. This difference was largely due to the care practices and operational policy of the two residences.

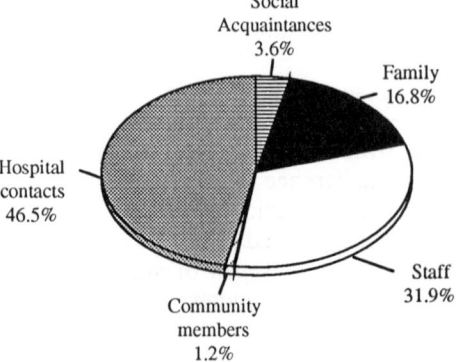

Community Care Scheme 1

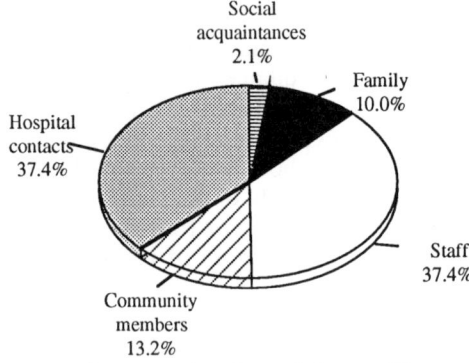

Community Care Scheme II

Figure 5.1 Pie charts indicating distribution of network membership at two community care schemes

These care practices are discussed in greater detail in chapter 3 Scheme I had 10 staff on duty during the week on a rotational basis. However, Scheme II had five staff per house, with the extra possibility of two management staff coming in weekly.

Interestingly, individuals in Scheme II reported more community members than those in Scheme I. Indeed, by comparison it can be seen that Scheme I residents reported very few community members in their networks. This was surprising as shops and local amenities were much more accessible to Scheme I than to Scheme II. However after investigation of care philosophy and care practices, it was found that in Scheme I individuals' time was very much their own and was less structured. In Scheme II time was more structured by staff around domestic chores.

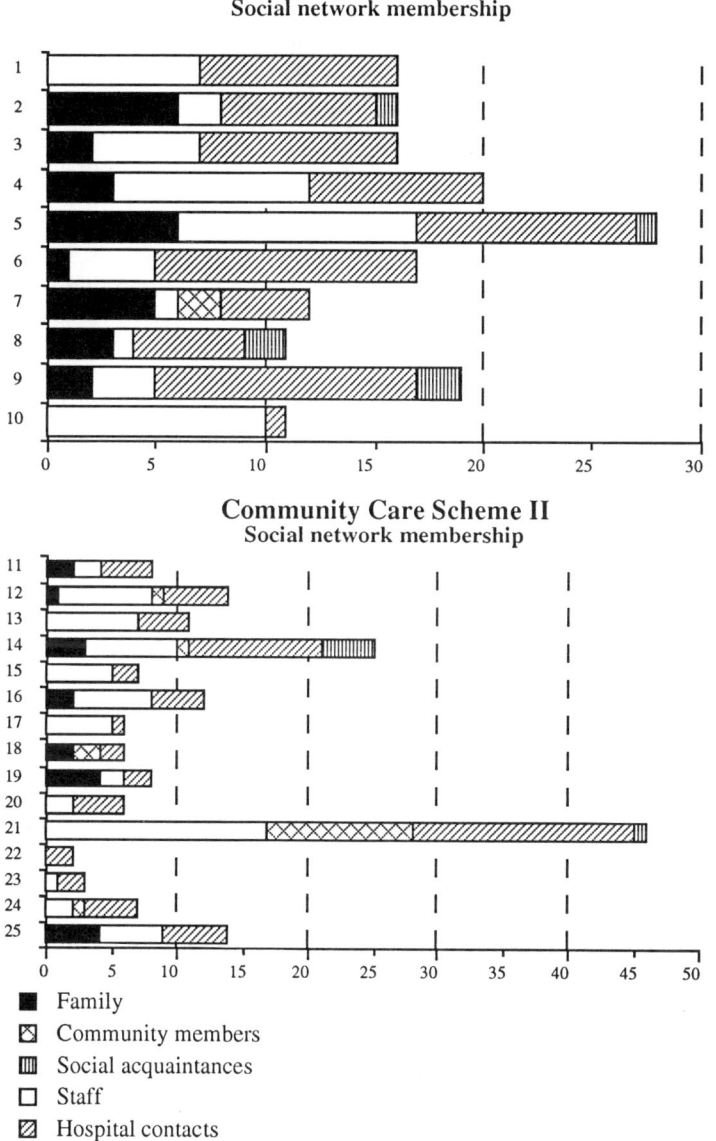

Figure 5.2 Network membership for individuals by community care scheme

This meant that residents would accompany staff when shopping, getting pensions and so forth. This was often followed by an outing to a local cafe where individuals were commonly known by name. In these regards, it could be said that contacts with community members were mediated very considerably by the care practices adopted by staff.

In both care schemes contacts originating in hospital were the most prevalent with an average of 5.8 members. However, of this total, individuals in Scheme I saw more hospital contacts than those in Scheme II. This could be accounted for by the fact that there were ten residents who had moved from hospital sharing Scheme I. In particular, residents tended to sit in the communal lounge for at least part of the day. Furthermore, Scheme I was within walking distance of the North Wales Hospital. Some individuals would often return to the wards and see 'old mates'. Two residents still worked in the hospital gardens. This provided another opportunity to keep in contact with 'old friends'. Moreover, many individuals from the hospital were discharged to various homes and hostels in and around the North Wales town. It was therefore more likely that they would come into contact with each other in the town. Local cafes and public houses in particular proved to be common meeting grounds.

However, this was not always viewed positively by residents. Some reported that they wished to meet up with people other than those from the hospital. In one or two cases individuals expressed strong desires to avoid any association with former hospital residents because they felt no affinity for them. Difficulties in shedding some features of institutional behaviour sometimes led to rejecting responses which could affect support network formation. For example, some residents became 'known' by locals for social behaviour which was not viewed as acceptable. This in turn sometimes precluded their participation in activities such as having a drink in a cafe. A case in point was a resident in Scheme I who chain smoked with small short inhalations without stopping to flick the ash until he had smoked the whole cigarette. This led the proprietors of the local café to ask him to leave the premises and to return only when he had finished his cigarette.

Few social acquaintances were named by individuals. This may be explained by the fact that individuals in Scheme II tended to engage in congregate activity in the company of staff, even when they went into the community. This restricted the formation of natural relationships. There was one exception to this. One individual named four people he had met in the church choir. In Scheme I individuals were given much more personal autonomy and many used this by venturing into town by themselves. They more often than not ended up in local cafes or public houses and it was here that they made their acquaintances.

To summarise, the data on membership indicates that after six months in the community, residents appeared to have made few new social contacts. Nineteen residents recorded no contacts with community members or social acquaintances. Rather, individuals were still principally in contact with people connected to psychiatric services. Although there has been little progress towards the social integration of people in local communities six months after they had been relocated, dislocation of friendships formed during hospitalisation appears to have been minimal. Six months after discharge, however, is still a relatively short time period upon which to make conclusive judgements about network formation and adjustment.

Qualitative data

The main purpose of using qualitative methods was to move towards an understanding of how individuals attribute meanings to relationships, and how they construe relationships with others in their social networks. Interviews were designed to provide an opportunity for individuals to present their own perceptions of the kinds of relationships they experienced. Informal questioning involved asking residents to express which members in their social networks were meaningful to them, what types of support the relationships provided, and the importance of these helping behaviours. Since the qualitative data revealed three principal membership categories, these were used as headings to record what relationships with these members appeared to mean for individuals.

Participant observation within the community over a seven month period began six months after hospital discharge. This made it possible to obtain a detailed picture of the types and sources of support received by residents, and to learn something about how these supportive relationships were experienced. Support in this context was classified as help offered to individuals in any sphere of their life which they found important. It was also the intention to find out if residents actively participated within their social networks, and specifically whether or not they provided help to others. Underlying this was an interest in understanding the nature and extent of exchange relationships within the study sample. The account that follows has been kept deliberately brief and merely gives an initial glimpse of how residents construed support.

Staff and social support

The data from interviews and observations showed that, on average, each resident had five staff members in their network, although as we have seen there were large individual differences. What then did these members mean to the individual?

It was found that, generally, direct care staff were significant in providing domestic help to residents. This largely took the form of shopping, cleaning and other domestic chores for those in Scheme II. Most residents living in Scheme II perceived project workers as 'nursing staff' to help run the house. The view was that this was nothing less than part of their job. Very few residents reported that there was anything more than just a care-giver relationship with staff, suggesting that the relationship was formal but functional for them.

For individuals living in Scheme I domestic help was encased within social activities. Residents were much more likely to see domestic help as a form of socialising. Domestic help was therefore not just the receiving of a meal on the plate - it was construed as a social event in itself. Similarly, personal care by project workers was construed as having far greater significance than a mere physical act. The intimacy involved appeared to generate relationships that came to be seen in terms of friendships.

Although staff members within individuals' networks were the main providers of domestic support and personal care, there were differences to be observed between care schemes and between individuals. This may be explained by the existence of different care philosophies and practices between the two schemes. In Scheme II, project workers were caring for three residents 24 hours each day in the closed environment of an ordinary house. Routine was based around domestic chores and in practice most of the staff actually did the work themselves with little involvement from residents. This was partly attributable to the age of the residents and the nature of their disabilities which made it difficult for some of them to participate. However, in Scheme I, the philosophy was one of enabling rather than providing. Residents were given a certain amount of encouragement to do things for themselves with staff just giving a hand here and there. In practice, residents were given the freedom to adopt lifestyles very much of their choice and so individuals who wanted to seclude themselves within the house could do so if they wished. A de-emphasis on active intervention was to mean that social relationships between residents and significant others were not actively fostered by staff members.

To summarise this brief characterisation of contacts with staff, it could be said that residents tended to report experiences largely in terms of instrumental support, although it was noted that some residents conceived of this support as taking place within relationships where there was a close emotional affinity or friendship between themselves and staff. The degree and type of engagement with residents appeared to be premised on contrasting philosophical approaches to care between the two community care schemes.

There is the possibility that residents are only partially aware of the more invisible components of caring or support roles such as that entailed in anticipatory and preventive care which some writers contend are often overlooked when care is being conceptualised (Bowers 1987). For example, surveillance, monitoring of drug compliance or side effects and many other caring tasks can be carried out in a relatively covert manner intended to minimise the awareness amongst residents that this was happening at all. Often the aim in such instances is to reinforce an image of independence and high self- esteem amongst residents. The perceptions of staff about their roles and tasks however are beyond the scope of this paper.

Family and social support

It was shown earlier (Table 5.2) that membership of support networks by family varied quite sharply between the two care schemes. Residents in Scheme II, being much older and having experienced twice the length of hospitalisation than their colleagues at Scheme I, named far fewer family members in their networks. Eight of the 15 residents at Scheme II and 2 of the 10 residents at Scheme I had no contact with any kin. The two residents in Scheme I who had no contact with kin had very different attitudes about this. Jane desperately wanted to see her brother, niece and nephew. She felt that the fact that they did not contact her meant that they did not think of her '...my brother, he never thinks of me... I've got no one'. The second resident did not especially want contact for reasons to do with perceptions about their present home:

> ...I've got four brothers...eh, they know where I am, you know, I'm not pushing it to see 'em you know...it's not important to keep in touch with them...you see, they've got their own lives to live and I've got my life. I don't want them coming down and seeing me here...because its degrading. I think so anyway...a place like this, I don't have to be in a place like this.

Seven out of the remaining eight residents in Scheme I did not wish to have contact with family members. The main reason for this appeared to be that kinship relationships had broken down at some point through the course of the illness and consequent upon the individuals' admission to hospital. The comments above suggest that some residents retain an acute sense of stigma about having been hospitalised and in residential care, which may account for their reluctance to maintain active social ties with family and relatives. Even though residents were now living in 'ordinary' housing in the community there was still a reluctance to renew contact with kin. The authors were unsure as to whether or not residents still associated the new housing with hospitalisation or whether too much time had elapsed for kin relationships to be reactivated. It seemed more likely that with the passage of time individuals had learnt to cope with the absence of kin and so no longer felt the need to have them as members in their network.

For the 15 residents who maintained contact with their families and relatives three means of contact were in evidence: visits, letters and telephone calls. In Scheme I, of those who were in contact with kin, four out of eight residents received family visits although only one resident had regular visits weekly. Five out of eight had to take the initiative and visit their kin. Another individual had visits from his aunt and uncle fortnightly. In Scheme II, six out of eight individuals received visits from their relatives. Therefore, in total ten out of fifteen residents had visitors. This showed that although extended kin had not totally rejected the individuals, visits were relatively infrequent. Some relatives were more prepared to visit individuals now that they were out of hospital. As stated by a member of staff, 'they (siblings) wouldn't visit him in hospital but they do now'.

Thus, most of the residents had to take the initiative if they wanted face-to-face contact with kin. Those who valued family contact were often not content with this. This ties in with related quality of life research (Barry and Crosby, 1992) which found that a relatively high percentage of residents going through the resettlement process, 27% at 12 months post-discharge, were dissatisfied with family contact. Although relatives of individuals in the study were more likely to phone and write letters than visit, residents still tended to take the initiative. Nevertheless, this tended to be restricted to Christmas and Birthdays so the level of contact through these means was very infrequent. Only two residents had phone calls from 'immediate' kin (both mothers) once a week or more often. Residents reported that such letters and phone calls were important to them in that they conveyed the sense that someone 'cared for them'. For the individuals concerned this shows that phones and letters can enable relationships to be active and intimate over long distances (Bell, 1968).

Material aid from family members was the only supporting behaviour reported by the residents. The literature on 'ordinary' social networks tends to suggest that even though kin may be separated by distance, financial aid can still be a predominant helping behaviour (Wenger, 1984). In the present study however only three residents reported financial assistance as a helping behaviour. As one of the three commented:

> My sister in Pembrokeshire is a widower. She is important to me because she helps me financially...she is very kind at Christmas and Birthday...she sends me tobacco.

Thus, material or financial help for individuals was again limited. This may well be due to the fact that extended kin do not have the same sense of obligation as close family members.

In summary, residents displayed a wide range of attitudes about contact with family members from unfulfilled expectations to ambivalence and outright rejection. One or two individuals eschewed the idea of family and relatives visiting because of anxieties about the stigma of living somewhere designated as a place for former psychiatric hospital residents. Visiting by family and relatives was uncommon for most residents, as well as being infrequent, and it was noted that much of the initiative about making contact was left to residents. Use of phones and letters nevertheless allowed some contacts to be maintained over long distances. Support from family members was therefore seen in more symbolic than practical terms.

All of the individuals were relocated into community settings with people that they had known in hospital. This invariably meant that they had known each other for a long period of time. The question arose of what meanings such ties had for individuals, especially now that they were sharing the same houses or flats.

Companionship appeared to be the main value that individuals attributed to their relationships. At one level companionship manifested itself in the form of conversations between residents but it could also involve passive behaviour such as just 'sitting' next to one another. It was not uncommon to see residents sitting together in the communal lounge of Scheme I as well as the lounges in the Scheme II houses saying very little to one another, while they watched television or listened to the radio. This type of behaviour shows that shades of institutionalism are still apparent despite the new community settings. It was akin to patterns of behaviour found by Dunn et al., (1990) who categorised residents' friends as 'patients who have a well defined group of companions with whom they spend their time, sitting, chatting and drinking tea, although often with long periods in silence'.

In the present study, conversations tended to centre around cigarettes, teasing or reminiscing about the 'old days' in hospital. Experiences of hospital life had taken up a very large part of individuals' lives and it appeared that this common bond was responsible for holding them together as a group of companions. However, when the researcher talked to individuals away from the group, it would often emerge that they did not wish to be associated with 'ex-psychiatric patients'. For example:

> a lot of people in ....I can't communicate with you know, they're in a world of their own, they're on medication, they're on drugs, they're out of their heads you know...

This suggests that individuals can harbour feelings of ambiguity or distancing towards other residents. On the one hand, such relationships offer solidarity through past and present experiences but on the other hand they put into question the development of new social relationships and therefore integration and participation within the wider community (Barham and Hayward 1991:55).

All of the individuals had their own rooms and in Scheme I each flat contained a lounge with a television. Thus, if they wanted to, individuals could spend time on their own or entertain guests. However, this was not construed as a preferred option. Rather, they chose to sit in the lounge. This was not necessarily a positive preference but was more a reaction to the fact that no structured activities were available.

'Having enough money' was not only important for everyday existence, but also for participating in the community. Being financially dependent upon state benefits, residents had little disposable income and this heavily circumscribed the activities in which they could participate. This was compounded by the fact that for many residents who were chain smokers most money was spent on cigarettes. Those in Scheme I in particular found that poverty was a major block to their participation in the community. This was noted by Barham and Hayward (1991) who described how individuals felt restricted in their 'social horizons'. Residents in Scheme I were usually given money for housekeeping purposes such as purchasing food and basic commodities but there was a tendency to spend a good deal of this to feed their smoking habit. A common scene in the lounge was residents asking staff and each other for money. Staff were prevented by contract from offering money to residents which left residents bartering with one another. One resident also occasionally begged from locals in the community to 'lend me a penny'. This kind of activity also represented the continuation of behaviour learnt in hospital. Interestingly, little was done by staff to extinguish this behaviour. The philosophy of Scheme I incorporated the idea that individuals would have to 'learn by experience' how to behave in the community. In this respect, the prevailing ethos could be construed as embodying a laissez-faire approach which emphasised the rights of individuals to self-determination.

Smoking, and the exchange of cigarettes, thus became a way in which residents could help each other. It also provided the basis of affinity with staff who smoked. A common sight was residents anticipating when staff or other residents needed to light a cigarette. This was observed to be the most prevalent form of reciprocal support between individuals within the study, confirming one of the central findings of the TAPS studies (Dunn, et al., 1990).

The giving and selling of cigarettes appeared to reflect patterns of dominance within relationships. When one individual had cigarettes and could actually supply another with them then they assumed some kind of leadership position. There was also an unwritten pressure to supply each other with cigarettes. This seemed to be exaggerated by the fact that cigarettes were one of the few items that individuals could offer one another. Thus in the absence of developed relationships, the exchange of cigarettes became very significant. It formed or made a statement about how or what the relationship was.

However, at Scheme II, the 'giving up' of smoking was regarded as a social progression as well as a healthy option. Therefore, as a matter of care practice, the supply of matches was restricted. Staff generally kept hold of cigarettes and would give them out to residents on a controlled basis. There was not the exchange relationship here. Rather, the behaviour was very much one-directional. Consequently, in some houses, residents would continually walk around with a cigarette in their hand asking for a light.

Apart from the exchange of cigarettes the buying of tea for one another was an important means of exchange between individuals, in particular for those living in Scheme I. Such behaviour was reminiscent of that observed in the coffee bar at the hospital during the pilot study. The exchange of tea and cigarettes was also found by Dunn, et al., (1990) to serve a social function for this long-stay population equivalent to that of conversation in other social groups.

Summarising the character of interpersonal relationships between residents is not easy because of the multi-stranded nature of many ties and connections between individuals, most of whom, in this case, have lived together for many years. Present behaviour was in this sense seen to be very much a product of historical ties between individuals. Hospital relocation strategy appeared to have recognised the importance of friendship networks between residents and these had to a large degree been preserved. Nevertheless it was observed that a good deal of the companionship consisted of passive activity or of behaviour which had an 'institutional' character. Relative poverty was raised as a constraint upon engagement in community-based activities. Living within small group settings was a preferred option for almost all residents but there was a sub-group who preferred not to associate with other residents on account of their wish to escape the common identity of having been a part of the psychiatric hospital system.

Discussion

It has been demonstrated that, overall, social network membership for this group is much more restricted in scale than that for other population groups or elderly population samples (Wenger, 1984). This supports previous psychiatric studies which found similar results (Dunn, et al., 1990; Thornicroft and Breakey, 1991). There is indirect evidence to suggest that for older individuals this is probably the result of kinship losses through death or family moves. That is, it arises as a result of family life-cycle processes. However, in numerical terms, kin were shown not to be the dominant members of individuals' networks. This was a position occupied by other residents and staff respectively. Indeed, beyond these membership groups there was little evidence that other persons entered into individuals' social networks at all. Six individuals out of the 25 accounted for all the community members in people's networks. Similarly, six individuals accounted for all the passing acquaintances that individuals could recall. This having been said, despite the restricted scale of individual' social networks there was considerable variation in network size between individuals.

Although, at the time of fieldwork, residents had been living in their neighbourhoods for at least six months (over 12 months by the end of fieldwork), few had developed any new relationships. A longitudinal follow up study is necessary to establish whether community-embedded relationships emerge. For the time being it is nevertheless gratifying to record that relocation has not resulted in dislocation of people's social contacts. Although it was not possible to begin the network study before individuals were discharged from hospital the social network data suggest that individuals comprising people's networks were much the same as they were when they were resident in hospital. This was partly the result of hospital discharge policy which sought to maintain friendship networks between individuals as they were moved from hospital. Put another way we could say that community presence (O'Brien and Lyle, 1989) has been achieved but that community participation, as expressed in the form of new social relationships with community members, is yet to become manifest.

From drawing some incidental comparisons between the two community care schemes it was noticeable that Care Scheme I adopted a more laissez-faire approach to the support of residents with the result that individuals were more free to exercise autonomy without structures being provided by staff. The idea therefore that people's social networks would grow 'naturally' or by some process of osmosis when they were moved to community settings after spending lengthy periods in hospital is not supported by the findings of this study. However, Figure 5.1 shows that by percentage, Scheme II residents had more community members in their networks than their peers in Scheme I. This appeared to be closely related to a distinctive pattern of care practices in the houses. Care staff felt a strong attachment to residents and were seen to adopt quasi- family roles in their direct work with residents. They actively participated in taking residents out into the community, often facilitating introductions to community members. There was some evidence to suggest that some meaningful new relationships developed in this way. The paradox is that the older, initially more disabled individuals in the sample (Scheme II) had been enabled to make more progress in this respect than their Scheme I counterparts. This suggests that individuals with a long history of mental illnesses and institutionalisation need staff support to gain access to the wider social context within which they live. Expecting people to initiate their own relationships would not appear to be a favoured method for promoting the social integration of individuals in the community. Indeed it may well put them at risk and expose them in an unprotected way to the more predatory instincts of some members of the community.

However, one of the concomitants of the process of movement from hospital to community settings appears to be that particular institutional behaviours from the past still continue. The existence of a sub-culture whose rules are governed by the exchange and bartering of cigarettes was very much in evidence, although steps were being taken at the Scheme II houses to de-emphasise such behaviour. The persistence of this behaviour typifies some central dilemmas for practitioners and policy makers: exchange and bartering of cigarettes is central to the maintenance of reciprocal relationships between many individuals and provides a basis for the learning of social skills. On the other hand reciprocal relationships between residents appeared hardly to exist on other levels so the exchange element seems to have a functional utility limited almost solely to cigarettes. The use of cigarettes gave individuals something to bargain with and for some individuals it seemed to be one of the few ways in which they could exercise a sense of personal leadership or initiative in their lives, whilst also contributing a feeling of solidarity in a common predicament. On the other hand it was a common predicament from which some individuals wanted escape. It may also be argued that since there was often very little for residents to do with their time and even less opportunity for individuals to engage in meaningful employment or activity, then this further restricted communication between individuals which can lead to the formation of relationships.

Overall it has been shown that whilst social networks were found to be relatively impoverished in relation to size, this was far from true for everyone. Membership details illustrated, however, that persons connected to mental health services dominate people's networks. The brief descriptions offered of how residents construed their relationships with different categories of network members showed that there were different and, at times, conflicting value positions assumed by residents about what they wanted from relationships with staff, other residents and family and relatives. This suggests that staff roles need to be appraised in terms of how they might best accommodate the supports, conflicts and controls (House, Umberson and Landis, 1988) which emerge from an appreciation of how social relationships and social networks impinge on people's lives.

It is important to stress that the findings reported remain tentative owing to the relatively short time spent by residents in the new community settings. However, the findings suggest the existence of a link between service processes, particularly care practices and philosophy, and outcomes, at least as expressed in the membership of residents' social networks and how relationships with categories of network members were construed. If one of the goals of policy is to facilitate a shift from community presence to community participation, then care staff will need clearer guidance and support in identifying community resources, in developing effective strategies to harness those resources to support the identified needs of individuals, in helping residents to come to informed choices about the use of those resources, and in evaluating outcomes as an integral part of the care process. It is possible that an applied social network analysis of the kind adopted in this study if incorporated into care practices, would help to sensitise care staff to the potential for helping residents to lead more socially integrated lives. The starting point, however, has to be an appreciation of those needs and wants as expressed by residents themselves. This would suggest that policy needs to be able to strike a balance between, on the one hand, extremes of social over-protection and, on the other hand, complete freedom and autonomy for residents. Striking the right balance can clearly be elusive. It is to be hoped, in the interests of residents, that it will not remain elusive for long.

References

Anderson, J., Dayson, D., Wills, W., Gooch, C., Margolius, O., O'Driscoll, C. and Leff, J. (1993), 'The TAPS Project 13: Clinical and Social Outcomes of Long-Stay Psychiatric Patients After One Year in the Community', *British Journal of Psychiatry*, 162 (suppl. 19),, 45-56.

Anderson, M. (1980), *Approaches to the History of the Western Family 1500-1914*. Hampshire, Macmillan Publishers Ltd.

Baker, R. and Hall, J.N. (1983), *Users' Manual for Rehabilitation Evaluation*. Aberdeen, Vine Publishing Limited.

Barham, P. and Hayward, R. (1991), *From the Mental Patient to the Person*. London and New York, Tavistock/Routledge.

Barry, M.M. and Crosby, C. (1992), 'Community Mental Health Care: Promoting a Better Quality of Life for Long-Term Clients'. Proceedings of Keele Conference, 1992. Promotion of Mental Health,2.

Bell, C.R. (1968), *Middle Class Families*, Routledge and Kegan Paul, London.

Bowers, B.J. (1987), 'Inter-generational Caregiving: Adult Caregivers and their Aging Parents', *Advances in Nursing Science*, 9, 2, 20-31.

Bronfenbrenner, U. (1979), *The Ecology of the Human Development Experiments by Nature and Design*. Cambridge, MA: Harvard University Press.

Brown, G.W., and Harris, T. (1978), *Social Origins of Depression: A Study of Psychiatric Disorders in Women*. New York, Free Press.

Bulmer, M. (1987), *The Social Basis of Community Care*. London, Allen and Unwin.

Cohen, C.I. and Sokolovsky, J. (1978), 'Schizophrenia and social networks: ex-patients in the inner city', *Schizophrenia Bulletin*, 4, 4, 565-560.

Crittenden, P.M. (1985), 'Social Networks, Quality of Child Rearing and Child Development', *Child Development,* 56, 1299-1313.

D'Abbs, P. (1982), *Social Support Networks: A Critical Review of Models and Findings.* Melbourne, Institute of Family Studies Monograph No 1.

Dayson, D. (1992), 'The TAPS project 15: The social networks of two group settings: a pilot study', *Journal of Mental Health,* 1, 99-106.

Dunn, M., O'Driscoll, C., Dayson, D., Wills, W., Leff, J. (1990), 'The TAPS Project 4: An Observational Study of the Social Life of Long-Stay Patients', *British Journal of Psychiatry,* 157, 842-848.

Dunst, C.J. and Trivette, C.M. (1988), 'Toward Experimental Evaluation of the Family, Infant and Preschool Program', in H.B. Weiss and F.H. Jacobs (eds), *Evaluating Family Programs.* New York, Aldine.

Dunst, C.J., Trivette, C.M. Gordon, N.J. and Pletcher L.L (1989), 'Building and Mobilizing Informal Family Support Networks.', in Singer G.H.C. and Irvin L.K. (eds), *Support for Caregiving Families: Enabling Positive Adaptation to Disability.* Baltimore, Paul H Brookes.

Fisher, J.D., Nadler, A. and DePaulo, B.M. (eds), (1983), *New Directions in Helping: Recipient Reactions to Aid.* New York, Academic Press.

Gottlieb, B.B. (ed), (1981), *Social Networks and Social Support.* Beverly Hills, London, Sage Publications.

Gourash, N. (1978), 'Help Seeking: A Review of the Literature', *American Journal of Community Psychology,* 6, 5, 413-23.

Grant, G. and Wenger, G.C. (1993), 'Dynamics of Support Networks: Differences and Similarities Between Vulnerable Groups', *Irish Journal of Psychology,* 14, 1, 79-98

Henderson, S. (1977), 'The Social Network, Support and Neurosis: The Function of Attachment in Adult Life', *British Journal of Psychiatry,* 131, 185-91.

Henderson, S., Byrne, D.G., Duncan-Jones, P., Scott, R., and Adcock, S. (1980), 'Social Relationships, Adversity and Neurosis: A Study of Associations in a General Population Sample', *British Journal of Psychiatry,* 136, 574-583.

HMSO (1991), *Standard Occupational Classification Volume 3. Social Classifications and Coding Methodology.* London, HMSO.

House, J.S., Umberson, D. and Landis, K.R. (1988), 'Structures and Processes of Social Support', *Annual Review of Sociology,* 14, 293-318.

Knapp, M., Cambridge, P., Thomason, C., Beecham, J., Allen, C. and Darton, R. (1992), *Care in the Community: Challenge band Demonstration.* Aldershot, Ashgate.

Leff, J. (ed), (1993), 'The TAPS Project: Evaluating Community Placement of Long-Stay Psychiatric Patients', *British Journal of Psychiatry,* Vol. 162. Supplement 19.

O'Brien, J. and Lyle, C. (1989), *Framework for Accomplishments.* Georgia, Responsive Systems Associates.

133

Pattison, E.M, DeFrancisco, D., Ward, P., Frazier, H. and Crowder, J. (1975), 'A Psychosocial Kinship Model for Family Therapy', *American Journal of Psychiatry*, 132, 1246-1251

Pilisuk, M. and Froland, C. (1978), Kinship, Social Support and Health. Social Science and Medicine, 128, 273-280.

Rook, K.S. (1992), 'Detrimental Aspects of Social Relationships: Taking Stock of an Emerging Literature', in Veiel, H and Baumann. U. (eds), *The Meaning and Measurement of Social Support*. New York, Hemisphere.

Sarason, I.G., Levine, H.M., Basham, R.B., Sarason, B.R. (1983), 'Assessing Social Support: The Social Support Questionnaire', *Journal of Personality and Social Psychology*, 44, 1, 127-139.

Smith, G. and Cantley, C (1985), *Assessing Health Care: A Study in Organisational Evaluation*. Milton Keynes, Open University.

Sokolovsky, J., Cohen, C., Berger, D. and Geiger, J. (1978), 'Personal Networks of Ex-Mental Patients in a Manhattan SRO Hotel', *Human Organization*, 37, 1, 5-15.

Taylor, R.D.W., Huxley, P.J. and Johnson, D.A.W. (1984), 'The Role of Social Networks in the Maintenance of Schizophrenic Patients', *British Journal of Social Work*, 14, 129-140.

Thornicroft, G. and Breakey, W.R. (1991), 'The COSTAR Programme. 1:Improving Social Networks of the Long-Term Mentally Ill', *British Journal of Psychiatry*, 159, 245-249.

Walker, K.N., MacBride, A., and Vachon, M.L.S. (1975), 'Social Support Networks and the Crisis of Bereavement', *Social Science and Medicine*, 11, 35-41.

Wallace, C.J. (1984), 'Community and Interpersonal Functioning in the Course of Schizophrenic Disorders'. *Schizophrenia Bulletin*, 10, 233-257.

Weiss, R.S. (1969), 'The Fund of Sociability', *Transactions*, 6, 36-39.

Weiss, R.S. (1974), 'The Provisions of Social Relationships', in Rubin, D. (ed), *Doing Unto Others*. New Jersey, Prentice-Hall.

Wenger, G.C. (1984), *The Supportive Network: Coping with Old Age*. London, Allen and Unwin.

Whittaker, J.K. and Garbarino, J. (eds), (1983), *Social Support Networks: Informal Helping in the Human Services*. New York, Aldine Publishing Company.

Winik, L., Zetlin, A.G. and Kaufman, S.Z. (1985), 'Adult Mildly Retarded Persons and their Parents: The Relationship Between Involvement and Adjustment', *Applied Research in Mental Retardation*, 6, 409-19.

Yoder, J., Jonker, J. and Leaper, R. (1985), *Support Networks in a Caring Community*. Dordrecht, Martinus Nijhoff.

Young, M.D. (1962), *Family and Kinship in East London*. (revised edition), Baltimore, Penguine Books.

Zarling, C.L., Hirsh, B.J. and Landry, S. (1988), 'Maternal Social Networks and Mother-infant Interactions in Full-term and Very Low Birthweight Pre-term Infants', *Child Development*, 59, 178-185.

6 Assessing the impact of community placement on quality of life

Margaret M. Barry and Charles Crosby

Summary

This chapter examines the impact of community placement on the quality of life of long-stay residents being discharged from the North Wales Hospital. The development and implementation of a quality of life schedule for use with a long-stay population is described together with a discussion of the methodological and practical implications of using quality of life as an outcome measure. Drawing on the findings from the first research cohort, this chapter reports on the quality of life experienced by residents on the hospital wards prior to discharge and a comparison is made with the quality of life experienced by the same individuals up to one year following their move to community settings. A number of significant positive changes in quality of life are reported and clients are generally very positive about their life in the community.

The utility of quality of life as an evaluative framework against which to assess the outcomes of care are considered. The need for further development in the measurement of this concept for a chronic population is discussed both in terms of its theoretical and practical implications.

Introduction

The quality of life study set out to investigate the determinants of quality of life for long-stay residents being discharged from hospital and to examine how the resettlement process impacted on their perceived quality of life. Improved quality of life is now widely recognised as an explicit priority of the community alternatives to hospital-based care (Anthony, 1980; Bachrach, 1980; Shadish, Orwin, Silber, and Bootzin, 1985) and its importance as a desired outcome for care programmes for chronic psychiatric populations has been highlighted by a number of practitioners

137

and researchers in this area (Bachrach, 1980; Baker and Intagliata, 1982; Bigelow, Brodsky, Stewart and Olson 1982; Lehman, 1988; Sartorius, 1992). The extent to which community-based facilities can have a positive impact on the lifestyles of long-term clients and maximise their quality of life is an important test of the success of the new services in translating their policy objectives into practice. As such, quality of life along with indicators of clinical and social functioning, constitutes a critical outcome measure in the present evaluation study, seeking to determine the broader impact of resettlement on the lifestyles and well-being of discharged hospital residents.

Despite the emphasis afforded quality of life, reviews of the literature suggest that there is a paucity of studies detailing the patterns of clients' lives and the factors that contribute to overall quality of life following discharge from hospital. The experience of being discharged from hospital and re-entering the community has rarely been reported upon from the perspective of the clients (Murphy, 1991; Pinkey, Gerber and Lafave, 1991). The majority of evaluation studies that have been carried out tend to be service based giving limited information on the lives of the clients and their experiences once they have been discharged into the community. Jones, Robinson and Golightley (1986) call for detailed tracer studies which take the client rather than the service as the focus, giving a more detailed account of actual situations, patterns of existence, and the factors in the material and social environment, together with subjective life experiences that contribute to overall quality of life. There have been few studies of this type which have attempted to detail the patterns of clients' lives and to ascertain the clients' perspectives concerning their own discharge and their reactions to life in the community.

American studies of the quality of life of chronic clients living in the community point to the many social problems affecting their quality of life. Both Lehman, (1982, 1983) and Baker and Intagliata (1982) report that life areas such finance, unemployment, personal safety and health are consistent sources of dissatisfaction for chronic clients and that they generally report a lower quality of life compared to that of the general population. However, despite the problems reported by clients living in the community, the majority report satisfaction with being out of hospital and do not express a desire to return to hospital. Lehman, Possidente and Hawker (1986) compared the quality of life of chronic clients in a state hospital with that experienced by clients in supervised community residences. Lehman et al. found that hospital patients report a lower quality of life than clients living in the community and that in-patients and community residents differed most in their satisfaction with living situation. Simpson, Hyde and Farragher (1989) also report a number of deficiencies in relation to hospital-based care for chronic clients in Britain. Comparing the quality of life of chronic clients in an acute wards in a district general hospital, a hostel ward and group homes, Simpson et al. report that quality of life was lower on the hospital ward than in the other two settings and that lack of safety and comfort in the hospital setting seriously detracted from residents' quality of life.

The findings from these studies are limited, however, by the fact that the groups sampled were not randomly allocated to the different care facilities. Placement within certain types of facilities tends to correspond with the severity of psychopathology, and this may in turn affect the quality of the living environment, thereby confounding the validity of the findings. Also of importance is the fact that comparisons between groups do not allow for the influence of individual differences in perception of life quality in different care environments. However, the studies do place the findings from community-based care in a more balanced perspective and suggest that while the quality of life of chronic clients in the community may be problematic, traditional hospital care may not necessarily be a better option. Coid (1993) points out that while there is increasing public concern over the plight of deinstitutionalised psychiatric patients, the quality of life of those in hospital has received relatively little attention or systematic investigation.

There are few longitudinal studies which trace the impact on individual clients of being moved from an institutional setting to live in the community. Prospective longitudinal studies offer the possibility of determining more clearly the influence of different forms of care delivery on clients' quality of life and of identifying which elements of the care process are critical to ensuring a high quality of life. Okin, Dolnick and Pearsall (1983) and Gibbons and Butler (1987) followed up small groups of clients as they were discharged from hospital, evaluating the effect of the move from hospital on their perceived quality of life. On the whole clients reported significant positive changes in their quality of life, they preferred life in the community and did not want to return to the hospital wards.

Prospective longitudinal studies which trace the same clients as they move from hospital into community settings, allow a much more direct comparison of quality of life under different care regimes. Such prospective longitudinal studies will enable us to establish empirically whether appropriately designed community-based residences can succeed in enhancing the quality of life of clients over and above that offered by traditional hospital care. Longitudinal studies also have a number of advantages from a methodological point of view. If quality of life is to function as a valid outcome measure, capable of discriminating those life areas most affected by different forms of care delivery, it is vital that the measures can be reliably demonstrated as offering sensitive indicators of the impact on clients' well-being of changes in either internal state or external life circumstances. As the majority of quality of life studies have been cross-sectional in nature, there have been few longitudinal studies demonstrating the sensitivity of the quality of life measures as discriminant outcome measures of mental health care delivery. The present study provides an ideal opportunity for examining these issues within the context of hospital closure and the community placement.

Method

Design

The design of the quality of life study is in accordance with the overall design of the project (as described earlier in chapter 2 in this volume) permitting the collection of data from the same individuals at a number of points prior to and following discharge from hospital. The longitudinal design of the study is closely linked to the timing of the resettlement programme and can therefore examine how changes in residential setting and form of care delivery influence clients' perceptions of their quality of life. The collection of three baseline measures in the hospital prior to discharge permits a detailed examination of the quality of life experienced by residents on the hospital wards, and the three post-discharge measures at six weeks, six months and twelve months determine the specific changes in quality of life brought about as a result of the move to the community. The prospective follow-up of the same individuals, monitoring changes in the reported levels of well-being over time and with changing living conditions, allows a much more direct evaluation of the relative benefits of hospital and community care for the long-stay population in the present study.

Assessing the quality of life of a long-stay psychiatric population

Current methods of assessing the quality of life of psychiatric clients tend to rely largely on self-report measures of both objective and subjective indicators of well-being. The measures of quality of life in psychiatric populations have taken their lead from large-scale national surveys of quality of life in the USA (Andrews and Withey, 1976; Campbell, Converse and Rodgers, 1976). This approach to assessing quality of life involves assessing both global well-being and life quality in specific life areas and it incorporates subjective and objective indicators. Though the specific domains used to describe quality of life have varied, they tend to include life areas such as social and family relations, living situation, work, finance, leisure and health.

A number of quality of life schedules have been developed for use with chronic psychiatric populations. These measures include the Oregon Quality of Life Questionnaire (Bigelow et al., 1982), the Life Satisfaction Profile (Bartlett and Intagliata, 1985), and Lehman's Quality of Life Interview (Lehman, Ward and Linn, 1982). Lehman's scale is probably the most widely used scale in this area and its psychometric properties have been most extensively examined (Lehman, 1988).

Lehman's quality of life scale was used initially to provide a basic framework for assessing the quality of life of long-stay residents on the hospital wards. As Lehman's scale was originally developed for use with chronic clients living in the community, its use with a long-stay in-patient population necessitated adaptations in terms of question and response formats. Pilot interviews were carried out with a sub-sample of the hospital cohort in order to ascertain the feasibility of conducting the quality of life interviews. An important consideration for the present sample, many of whom were elderly and quite dependent, was keeping the interview questions as short as possible, and ensuring that the interview could be administered to the whole sample, including the less articulate residents. The wording of certain questions and response formats were modified in order to increase comprehensibility and ease of implementation. Lehman's 'delighted-terrible' scale, for example, was replaced initially by a three point satisfaction scale, later progressing to a five-point scale, ranging from 'very satisfied' to 'very dissatisfied' with a central point labeled 'uncertain'.

The adapted schedule retains the same basic structure as Lehman's original scale covering objective and subjective indices in nine life areas together with indices of general well-being. A number of open-ended questions are also included in the schedule in order to explore individual perceptions of significant life events and experiences, attitude to discharge, reactions to the move from hospital, and perceived comparisons of hospital and community life. Further details of the adaptation of the schedule and its psychometric properties may be found in Barry, Crosby and Bogg (1993).

Internal reliability of the modified schedule

As the modified schedule contains 96 items in all, which is substantially less than that contained in Lehman's original scale, it was important from the outset to demonstrate its internal reliability. Internal consistency reliability coefficients (Cronbach's Alpha) were computed for each of the objective and subjective life domain scores based upon the initial baseline interview with the hospital sample (see Barry, Crosby and Bogg, op. cit.). In all, 68 of the 96 items were included in the life domain composite indices.

As may be seen in Table 6.1, the majority of the scales have reliability coefficients greater than .60 suggesting that the composite indices are adequate for comparison purposes. The reliability of the objective indices compares quite favourably with those reported by Lehman (1988), while the reliability of the subjective indices tends to be somewhat lower. The reliability of the objective living scale is lower than the other scales (r = .55); however, it is noted that Lehman (1988) also reports reliability estimates of less than .50 for living objective sub-scales such as autonomy, privacy and influence.

Table 6.1
Internal consistency reliability estimates for subjective and objective life domain composite indices

Life Domain†	No. of Items	Cronbach's Alpha
Subjective Indices		
Living Situation	5	.63
Social Relations	3	.87
Family Relations	2	.60
Leisure	2	.68
Work	5	.83
Health	5	.68
Personal Safety	2	.63
Objective Indices		
Living Situation	5	.55
Frequency of Social Contacts	9	.66
Frequency of Family Contact	3	.64
Leisure Activities	13	.63
Physical Illness in Past Year	2	.95
Contact with Mental Health Professionals	5	.64

† Single item scales are not included in this table.

Data analysis

Analysis of the data was carried out on both the subjective and objective indices in each of the nine life domains. Composite indices were compiled by summing the scores of the individual items in each life area, thereby permitting sub-scores to be calculated for both the objective and subjective indices in each life domain. Given that the satisfaction items were scored at first interview using a three-point scale, the composite scores are based on summing the items in each domain rather than on the mean of the items.

Procedure

The quality of life interviews were carried out with each individual client by members of the research team in a private location out of ear shot of either hospital or community care staff. The quality of life interview was done in most cases in one sitting, usually at the same time as the psychiatric interview described earlier, and responses were considered generally reliable and valid. In addition to the interview schedule for clients, a list of questions concerning the objective indicators of life quality for each of the clients was also completed by a staff member, usually the client's key worker, in both the hospital and community placements. This information was obtained in order to cross check the reliability of data

142

derived from clients concerning objective indicators such as finances, health, frequency of family contact etc.

(The term 'patients' or 'hospital residents' will be used to refer to the study's sample while in the hospital setting while the term 'clients' will be used to refer to the sample once they have been discharged from hospital).

Baseline measures of quality of life in hospital prior to discharge

The quality of life interviews were carried out with 62 of the baseline sample of long-stay patients resident on the rehabilitation wards at the North Wales Hospital. As descibed in fuller detail in chapter 2, the majority of the sample (83%) had a clinical diagnosis of schizophrenia, ranged in age from 27 to 87 years (mean age = 56 years), had spent lengthy periods in hospital (mean total years in hospital = 25.6 years) and demonstrated low levels of social and behavioural functioning. In all three sets of interviews were carried out with each resident at three monthly intervals in the period prior to discharge. A more detailed description of the baseline findings and their implications may be found in Barry, Crosby and Mitchell (1992).

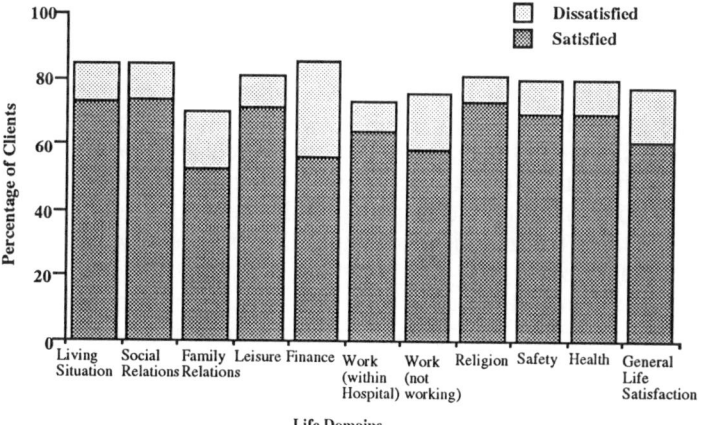

Figure 6.1
Hospital baseline levels of satisfaction: Domain-specific and general life satisfaction (N=62)

The main findings are summarised here. The initial baseline results revealed that the quality of life of hospital residents as measured by the objective indicators appeared to be severely restricted. Levels of independence and privacy on the hospital wards tended to be low, with low levels of interactive contact among the patients. The most frequent source of daily interaction was with staff, with 39% of patients reporting

143

not interacting socially with other patients on the ward. Many of the patients were socially isolated, with few sources of social support outside the hospital. Few patients engaged in active leisure activities, and none was in employment at the time of interview; however, 36% did carry out work within the hospital for which they received a small payment.

Despite the objective living conditions, self-reported levels of satisfaction were high in most life areas (see Figure 6.1), with the highest levels of satisfaction being reported in relation to social relations (73%), religion (73%) and living situation (72%). The life areas that elicited the highest levels of dissatisfaction were frequency of family contact (31% dissatisfied) and finance (29% dissatisfied). Hospital residents expressed a desire to receive more weekly spending money and were also keen to have more contact with their families. However, even in these life areas the majority appeared to be satisfied with their current life situation. Reports of general life satisfaction were also high (61%), but were somewhat lower than those expressed in the specific life domains.

Open-ended data

The open-ended questions explored hospital residents' perceptions of what was important in their lives, including sources of enjoyment and unhappiness, together with personal aspirations and hopes. Examination of the qualitative data suggested that many residents experienced some difficulty in responding to such questions. For example, 51% of the sample were either unable or unwilling to specify what was of most importance in their lives, (e.g. I don't think about it', 'cannot think of anything'), while 62% of the sample did not specify aspects of their lives they would like to change for the better, (e.g. 'too late now to think that, too late and not early enough'). For those who did respond, replies generally referred to the life areas covered by the interview schedule such as family, work, leisure and social relationships.

While these general life areas emerged as being of importance, aspects of the more immediate living environment were also perceived as salient determinants of life quality for this hospitalised group. In response to questions concerning sources of enjoyment or unhappiness, patients tended to refer to events in the immediate environment. For instance, complaints about the other patients or about hospital life in general were the most common sources of displeasure, while cigarettes, teas and coffees were cited as the most popular sources of enjoyment. Residents' expressed aspirations were quite low and many seemed resigned to life in hospital, (e.g. ' I'm in hospital and that's about it ', 'life is nearly over, things could have been better'').

With regard to attitude to discharge, the majority of clients (52%) did express a desire to leave the hospital, despite the fact that 42% were unsure if they would be better off as a result of the move. Attitude to discharge was found to be influenced by such factors as length of stay, with the older patients who had been hospitalised for lengthy periods tending to hold negative attitudes toward resettlement.

Stability of the baseline measures

The temporal stability of the quality of life indices was also ascertained by assessing the degree of change in the quality of life indices over time independent of significant changes in living circumstances. Repeated measures analyses were carried out on the three quality of life assessments in the hospital setting in order to determine the degree of fluctuation over over a six month period. The results, which are reported in detail in Barry, Crosby and Bogg (1993), showed that the quality of life indices were stable over the three assessment points, producing a stable baseline against which to assess the impact of community living on this long-stay population.

Interrelationship of quality of life indices

An analysis of the inter-correlations of the baseline quality of life indices revealed few significant findings (see Table 6.2). There was an absence of significant correlations between the majority of the subjective and objective indicators in each life domain. This finding is consistent with that reported in previous studies (Andrews and Withey, 1976; Campbell et al., 1976; Lehman, 1988). From the total set of correlations computed, only two emerged as significant: these were a positive correlation between satisfaction with social relations and frequency of contacts within the hospital ($r = 0.24$, $p < .05$), and a negative correlation between satisfaction with health and use of health care services ($r = -0.34$, $p < .05$).

Correlations between general life satisfaction and the domain-specific indicators were also carried out. Consistent with previous reports in the literature, the domain-specific subjective indicators were found to be significantly related to general life satisfaction. The strongest correlations were in the areas of social relations ($r = 0.61$, $p < .001$), living situation ($r = 0.57$, $p < .001$), and health ($r = 0.46$, $p < .001$).

However, the domain-specific objective indicators were not significantly correlated with reports of general life satisfaction.

The influence of demographic and clinical characteristics

The relationship between general life satisfaction and a number of demographic and clinical variables was also explored (see Table 6.3). Characteristics such as age and current length of hospital stay were not found to be correlated with reports of general life satisfaction. However, general life satisfaction was found to be correlated with levels of dependency and psychiatric functioning. A significant positive correlation was found between overall level of dependency, i.e. total general behaviour score as measured on the REHAB scale (Hall and Baker, 1983), and general life satisfaction (r = 0.23, p < .05). The more dependent patients were more likely to report higher levels of general life satisfaction than those who were more able and more independent. In relation to this finding, it is interesting to note the relationship between attitudes to discharge and general life satisfaction. The results showed that general life satisfaction correlated positively with a desire to remain in hospital (r = 0.38, p < .01), and was negatively correlated with positive expectations concerning discharge from hospital (r = -0.23, p < .05). This finding highlighted the need to consider the effects of institutionalisation on levels of expressed satisfaction in hospital, as high levels of expressed satisfaction may be simply reflecting patients' adaptation and resignation to a dependent and restricted life style. This finding has particular relevance in investigating the quality of life of long-term patients with high levels of dependency.

Table 6.2
Spearman correlations between subjective and objective indicators of quality of life at hospital baseline (N = 62) and at 12 months post-discharge (N = 29)

Subjective Indicator	Objective Indicator	Hospital Baseline	Community
Living Situation	Living Objective Measures	.06	.01
Social Relations	Frequency of Social Contacts	.06	-.03
	(b) Contacts within facility	.24*	.39*
	(c) Contacts outside facility	-.20	-.03
Family Relations	Frequency of Family Contacts	.16	.14
Leisure	Leisure Activities	-.08	.27
Finances	Weekly Spending Money	-.18	-.19
Health	Illness in Past Year	-.09	-.49**
	Use of Health Services	-.34*	.04*
Religion	Religious Practice	-.02	.46*
Safety	Victim of Attack	.03	.05

* p < .05; **p < .01

Two indices of psychopathology, as rated on the Brief Psychiatric Rating Scale (Overall and Gorham, 1962), were found to be significantly correlated with general life satisfaction; depression (r = -0.29, p < .05) and thought disorder (r = -0.53, p < .001). Hospital residents with higher ratings of depression and thought disorder were more likely to report lower levels of overall life satisfaction. Lehman (1983b), using the Rand Health Insurance Study Mental Health Battery as an index of psychopathology, reported significant negative correlations between general life satisfaction and anxiety and depression. However, Lehman did suggest that, 'It is conceivable that other measures of psychopathology might bear a different relationship to quality of life measures,...' (1983b, p.149). It is therefore interesting, in this context, to compare Lehman's findings with those found in the present study employing the Brief Psychiatric Rating Scale.

Table 6.3

Correlation of general life satisfaction with demographic and clinical characteristics at hospital baseline (N= 62) and at 12 months post-discharge (N = 29)

Variable	Spearman Correlation Coefficients	
	Hospital	Community
Age in Years	.19	-.10
Total Years Hospitalised	.12	-.07
Dependency Level		
(REHAB TGB score)	.22	-.13
BPRS Symptom Ratings		
Anxiety	-.06	-.26
Depression	-.29*	.04
Thought Disorder	-.53***	.03
Hallucinations	-.21	-.03
Conceptual Disorganisation	-.13	.08
Emotional Withdrawal	.14	.10
Blunted Affect	.10	.05

*p < .05; *** p <.001

Discussion and implications of the hospital findings

The findings from the hospital phase of the study showed the adapted version of Lehman's scale to be a viable instrument for use with a long-stay psychiatric population. The analysis indicated that the modified schedule has satisfactory psychometric properties, demonstrating adequate internal consistency reliability. Concerning the content validity of the schedule, the qualitative data from this study suggest that life areas such as family, social relations and leisure are indeed important to people with chronic psychiatric problems, thereby justifying their inclusion in the schedule. However, the importance of specific aspects of the individual's immediate environment to overall quality of life must not be overlooked, particularly in relation to a hospitalised or residential population. The results of the repeated measures analysis across the three assessment points showed that the quality of life measures are relatively constant over time providing evidence of a stable quality of life baseline against which to assess the impact of change of residence.

Consideration of the baseline results raised a number of methodological issues concerning interpretation of the findings and the validity of the measures used. A more detailed discussion of these issues may be found in Barry and Crosby (1994) and only the main points will be summarised here. The overall impression from the results is of a group of patients who rate low on quality of life as objectively measured, yet evaluate their subjective life quality in a positive manner. The lack of correlation between the two sets of indices raises a number of questions concerning how the data should be interpreted and how much weight should be given to each for evaluation purposes.

Regarding the objective quality of life indices, information obtained from care staff in the hospital concurred with the information derived from the patients which gives some confidence in the validity of reportage by patients. However, it is difficult to reconcile the discrepancy between the objectively low levels of quality of life and the high rates of expressed satisfaction. Studies of the life satisfaction of chronic psychiatric clients tend to report generally high levels of satisfaction, with the majority of clients reporting being 'mostly satisfied' in most life areas (Lehman, 1982; Baker and Intagliata, 1982). The subjective measures do, however, appear to be sensitive to the effects of psychopathology and dependency and, despite the clustering of positive responses, they succeed in highlighting areas where most dissatisfaction exists. However, the question does arise as to whether these high levels of expressed satisfaction should be accepted at face value as an expression of satisfaction with the current quality of life or whether they should be interpreted as an indication of dependency needs, a consequence of years of coping with disabling psychiatric problems.

These results suggest that the validity of the subjective measures requires closer scrutiny. Wilde and Svanberg (1990) point to reports of the biasing influence of such factors as social desirability effects (Carstenson & Cone, 1983) and acquiescent response set (Ware, 1978) on expressed satisfaction. Added to these difficulties for an in-patient population are the particular effects of institutionalisation and how a dependent lifestyle in hospital may lower levels of expectation and aspirations, leading residents to be content with a quality of life that many outside the hospital would consider unsatisfactory. The expectation gap between what someone has and what someone expects may be very narrow for institutionalised long-stay patients, giving rise to relatively high levels of satisfaction. The social comparison standards in operation in the hospital may therefore dramatically effect the whole process by which patients come to judge and appraise their life quality.

It is important that the issues raised above be taken into consideration when assessing the quality of life of people who have spent most of their adult life in a psychiatric institution, yet this aspect of the quality of life of a chronic psychiatric population is rarely addressed in the literature. The influence of institutional living and dependency on quality of life is an important finding in relation to the evaluation of residential psychiatric care, as these factors are likely to play an important role in determining how clients with a history of hospitalisation may come to assess the quality of life provided by residential community settings. The design of the present study permits an investigation of how the standards of comparison employed by individuals in their judgements of life quality will change as a result of greater exposure to different standards of living and social norms in the community. The influence of changes in psychiatric state, monitoring fluctuations in the levels of depressive and psychotic symptoms, and the effects of any changes in the level of dependency on reports of general well-being will also be considered. At a broader level, the influence of changes in residential setting, staff attitudes and operational policy on residents' quality of life must also be recognised. It is therefore important that the information derived from the quality of life schedule is related to these other outcome and process variables.

Perceived quality of life in the community settings

From the original hospital group, 34 were resettled into community residential facilities over the period of the study. A detailed description of the sample of hospital leavers and the community placements may be found in chapter 3 and 4. No significant differences were found between the baseline characteristics of 'leavers' and those who remained in hospital in terms of demographic and clinical characteristics such as age, length of stay, psychiatric state, overall level of functioning and attitude to discharge. It should be noted however, that in terms of the design of the present study, the repeated measures before and after discharge essentially means that the discharged group act as their own control in establishing the impact of community placement on their perceived quality of life. Follow-up interviews were carried out with those remaining in hospital in order to determine how their quality of life changed over the same time period. Therefore, due to attrition, completed quality of life interviews were carried out with 29 of the hospital leavers at twelve months post-discharge and with 15 of the hospital group awaiting discharge.

The adjustment to life in the community settings was monitored at six weeks, six months and twelve months following discharge from hospital. At each of the follow-up assessment points the discharged clients reported very favourable comments about their life in the community and a number of significant improvements in reported quality of life were already visible within six months of the move from hospital.

A more detailed account of the findings at six weeks and six months post-discharge respectively may be found in Crosby and Barry (1991) and Barry and Crosby (1993).

Although these early results were very encouraging, it was necessary to ascertain if initial positive outcomes would be maintained over at least a one year period. Perkins, Hollyman, Boardman, Humphreys-Hunt, Reeves and Weizmann (1992), in a one year follow-up of the functioning of long-stay clients resettled from hospital, warned of a 'honeymoon effect' which was found to last for about two months after resettlement, but then returned to pre-discharge levels. It is therefore important to monitor changes in clients' perceptions of quality of life as a function of their length of stay in the new community settings. A one year follow-up is regarded as a minimum period over which to monitor changes, particularly given the length of time many of the clients had spent in hospital before moving to the community.

Clients' reactions to life in the community

At each of the three post-discharge points clients' reactions to life in the community were extremely positive. Positive reactions were at their peak at six months post-discharge with 93% describing their lives in the community residences as being either much better (80%) or somewhat better (13%) than in hospital.

> 'generally happy' 'in everyway its better' 'I'm much happier here... my life has changed and I feel as if its a new life', ' They were too strict in hospital, your life wasn't your own, there's real freedom here',' I'm more independent, I can handle my own food and money, I can go shopping, self-medicate...'.

These positive reactions are quite significant given the fact that roughly one third of the discharged group, mainly the older clients, had not wanted to leave the hospital, but six months on, they report feeling much better for having made the move; 'I didn't want to move, but its much better here'. None of the clients express a desire to return to hospital. These positive comments were again in evidence at twelve months post-discharge. Though somewhat lower than that reported earlier in the study, the majority (72%) of clients described their lives in the community residences as being either somewhat better (3%) or much better (69%) than in hospital.

> 'Life is more ordinary now, I lived with 70 people before, I was in hospital too long', 'things are generally better here'

> 'a big improvement, things happen that make life more interesting - hobbies - I was bored in hospital, the staff are kinder here'

When questioned concerning which areas of their lifes were most affected by resettlement, the majority of the responses referred to the greater freedom and independence experienced by residents in the community settings;

> 'You've got more freedom to do what you want to do..' ' It's like having a home of my own... I can do anything any time I like, like shopping and cleaning. It's a big gain coming here' 'It's a better type of life altogether, there's freedom and happiness like I never had before'

150

Reported levels of satisfaction at twelve months post-discharge in comparison with hospital baseline levels for the discharged group are depicted graphically in Figure 6.2. Levels of satisfaction in each of the life domains ranged from 66 - 93 %, with highest levels of satisfaction being expressed in relation to living situation (93%) and social relations (90%). In particular, quite high levels of satisfaction were reported in relation to the privacy (100%), bedroom (97%), freedom (90%), accommodation (90%), and food (90%) provided by the community settings. The majority of clients express high levels of satisfaction with their relationship with the care staff (86%), the other clients (83%) and 62% report having friends within the care facility. Satisfaction with the treatment received in the community settings was also high, with 83% expressing satisfaction with the medical treatment and 83% satisfied with their opportunity to consult staff. Safety issues do not present as a problem with 86% of clients reporting satisfaction with personal safety in the community homes and 76% satisfied with safety in the neighbourhood. The glaring exception is satisfaction with religion which has dropped since moving to the community.

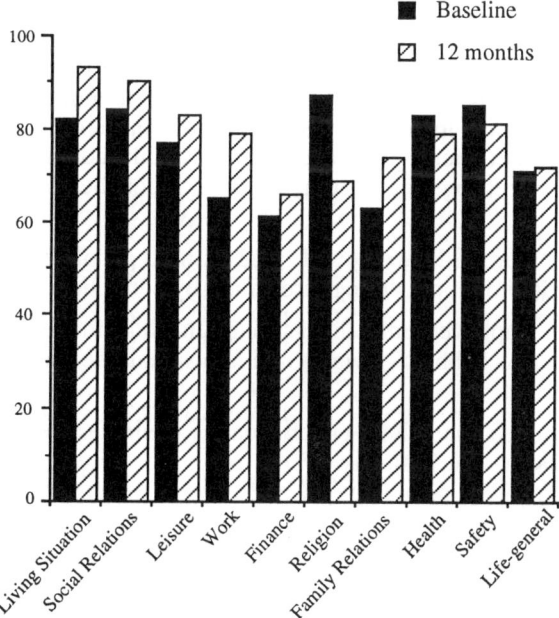

Figure 6.2
Satisfaction at hospital baseline and 12 months post-discharge in the community (N=29)

The lower rate of satisfaction is probably due to the fact that there was a chapel on the hospital grounds which hospital residents attended regularly and this routine has been lost since moving to the community.

The life areas that elicited the highest levels of dissatisfaction in the community were, amount of spending money available (31% dissatisfied), and frequency of family contact (28% dissatisfied). Clients express a desire to see their families more often with many wanting to live with family, even when this was not a feasible option. Levels of contact with family were not found to change appreciably following the move to the community, with 34% of community clients receiving family visits on at least a monthly basis compared to 39% of the hospital baseline sample. Expressed dissatisfaction with finances was generally accompanied by comments such as 'it all goes on food' , with little money left over for other personal expenses. The majority of the clients were satisfied with not having a job (79%) with many of the older clients feeling that they were 'too old for work now'. The dissatisfaction with not having a job was voiced mainly by the younger clients (10% dissatisfied) many of whom had been attending the hospital's industrial therapy unit. This service had not been replaced for clients within the first year of discharge and it would appear that some form of occupational or training activities would be of much benefit to the younger clients.

Table 6.4
Mean and SD life domain composite indices:
Repeat post-discharge assessments

Life Domain	6 weeks		6 months		12 Months		F Ratio
	M	SD	M	SD	M	SD	
Subjective Indices							
Living Situation	14.52	.87	14.40	.96	14.64	1.22	.30
Social Relations	9.00	.00	8.95	.21	8.64	1.05	2.23
Family Relations	5.06	1.69	5.12	1.67	5.25	1.44	.08
Leisure	5.48	1.00	5.52	1.00	5.44	1.00	.68
Finances	2.50	.93	2.46	.88	2.92	.95	.48
Religion	2.74	.69	2.69	.76	2.47	.85	1.07
Health		1.23	13.33	2.35	13.44	2.75	
Personal Safety	5.64	1.11	5.63	.85	5.32	1.25	.95
Objective Indices							
Living Situation	8.55	.95	8.80	.95	8.95	1.19	1.04
Social Objective	21.40	4.88	22.40	4.90	27.75	4.91	.99
Within the facility	10.83	2.44	11.30	2.90	11.48	2.92	.47
Outside the facility	5.27	2.55	5.95	2.77	5.59	2.59	1.46
Family Contact	5.48	2.82	5.52	2.71	6.09	2.74	1.35
Leisure Activities	18.81	2.27	20.38	2.38	20.43	2.54	7.95**
Weekly Money	18.38	14.43	27.67	22.04	17.10	14.84	4.47*
Physical Illness in Past Year	3.67	1.01	3.87	.45	3.83	1.09	.42
Frequency of Religious Practice	2.07	1.28	2.14	1.30	2.07	1.35	.06
Victim of Robbery	1.92	.28	1.80	.65	1.64	.49	2.29
Global	2.68	.75	2.80	.58	2.64	.70	.42

* p< .05; ** p< .01

Levels of general life satisfaction, however, were observed to drop from 87% at six months post-discharge to 72% at twelve months post-discharge, indicating a return to pre-discharge levels. This drop in global satisfaction may be indicative of a levelling off following an initial 'honeymoon effect' as suggested by Perkins et al. (op. cit.). Nevertheless, at twelve months post-discharge clients, in the present study continue to describe their lives as having improved following the move from hospital.

In order to assess the statistical significance of the changes in quality of life, repeated measures analyses of variance were carried out on the subjective and objective composite indices for each life domain. The means and standard deviations for the composite indices in each life domain across the three post-discharge assessment points are presented in Table 6.4. Analysis of variance with repeated measures (MANOVA) was carried out on each of the life domain scores for both the objective and subjective scales in order to check on the stability of the measures across the post-discharge data points. As can be seen from Table 6.4, there were no significant changes in the majority of the scales over the three post-discharge assessment points. With regard to the objective scales, reported levels of leisure activity were found to increase across the three data points (F = 7.95, p< .01). No other significant changes were found across the three post-discharge assessment points which indicate that, as in the hospital baseline phase of the study, the quality of life indices remain relatively stable. The presentation of the post-discharge findings will therefore focus on the analysis of the twelve months follow-up assessments.

Analysis was carried out on the subjective and objective composite indices for each life domain, comparing the hospital baseline findings for the 29 discharged clients with the quality of life reported at twelve months post-discharge. The results of the comparison between the hospital baseline findings for the discharged clients with their quality of life at twelve months post-discharge is presented in Table 6.5. Repeated measures analyses (MANOVA) of the subjective indices revealed a statistically significant improvement in relation to satisfaction with living situation, with clients reporting higher levels of satisfaction with their new residences in the community compared to the hospital wards (F = 6.94, p < .01). No other significant changes were found in the subjective indices. The increase in satisfaction with living situation was paralleled by a significant increase in the objective indices of living situation (F = 40.00, p< .001). Clients reported feeling comfortable in their new homes (93%), felt they belonged there (83%) and that they could decide when they wanted to do things for themselves (79%).

A number of significant changes also emerged in relation to social relations with increased social interaction in the community residences being reported by clients (F = 29.52, p < .01), both within the facility (F = 14.75, p < .01) and outside the facility (F = 5.02, p < .01). The main improvements to date appear to be in relation to higher levels of interactive contact among the clients and the care staff. The low rates of interaction among the clients in the hospital setting was commented on earlier in this chapter and in chapter 3 and it would appear that the more domestic-style dwellings in the community have facilitated increased levels of interaction.

Table 6.5
Mean (SD) life domain composite indices at hospital baseline and 12 months post-discharge in the community

| Life Domain | Hospital Baseline | | Community | | MANOVA |
	M	SD	M	SD	F Ratio
Subjective Indices					
Living Situation	13.39	2.39	14.61	1.20	6.94**
Social Relations	8.03	1.81	8.54	1.17	2.28
Family Relations	4.63	1.61	5.25	1.42	2.58
Leisure	5.25	1.08	5.54	.88	1.41
Finances	2.14	1.01	2.32	.94	.60
Religion	2.71	.76	2.43	.92	1.83
Health	13.16	1.93	13.40	2.50	.17
Personal Safety	5.37	1.11	5.30	1.24	.12
Objective Indices					
Living Situation	7.47	.92	8.80	1.01	40.00***
Frequency of Social Contacts	17.67	6.37	23.29	4.76	29.52**
Within the facility	8.44	3.90	11.48	2.61	14.75**
Outside the facility	4.88	2.93	5.82	2.96	5.02**
Frequency of Family Contact	5.43	2.73	6.19	2.90	2.49
Leisure Activities	19.20	2.81	20.31	2.47	3.79
Weekly Activities	13.07	1.98	13.88	1.67	4.57*
Yearly Activities	4.93	.99	5.00	1.00	.08
Finances	13.13	9.00	17.22	15.48	2.26
Physical Illness in Past Year	3.73	.67	3.77	1.11	.03
Frequency of Religious Practice	2.55	1.44	2.23	1.45	.70
Victim of Robbery/Attack	1.44	.51	1.63	.49	1.71
Global	2.39	.99	2.57	.74	.75

* $p < .05$; ** $p < .01$; *** $p < .001$

The increased level of social interaction outside the facility was mainly attributable to contact with other clients, either resident in another house in the resettlement scheme or still resident in hospital. The social network of the group appears to be made up, primarily, of contacts with care staff, family and other psychiatric clients. There are few reports of any new contacts being made since moving to the community. A significant increase was also found in relation to weekly leisure activities ($F = 4.57$, $p < .05$) with clients participating in more activities such as art and craft classes, and making greater use of local community facilities such as shops and cafes.

From the original research cohort 29 remained in hospital awaiting placement. Follow-up interviews were conducted with 15 of this group to examine any changes in their perceptions of quality of life over the time period of the study. Analysis was carried out comparing their baseline quality of life data with that reported at twelve months follow-up in the hospital. The results of the repeated measures analyses of variance (MANOVAs) reveal no significant differences in relation to the subjective indices. Only one of the objective scales showed significant improvements, an increase in weekly spending money ($F = 7.26$, $p < .05$). The objective living situation indices show a significant deterioration over the twelve month period ($F = 30.10$, $p < .001$). The assessment of the hospital living environments at baseline pointed to the lack of privacy, depersonalised living environment and lack of independence on the hospital wards (see Crosby et al., this volume). It would appear that patiens still in hospital awaiting discharge report a further deterioration in their living conditions. These reports were backed up by observations made by the researchers, noting a relative decline in conditions on the wards in the run up to hospital closure. The institutional environment of the hospital would appear to offer less in the way of independence and freedom for its residents in comparison with the community settings.

Interrelationship of quality of life indices at twelve months post-discharge

The relationship between the objective and subjective life domain scores was examined for the discharged group at twelve months post-discharge (see Table 6.2). As before, few significant correlations emerged; a significant positive correlation between satisfaction with social relations and the frequency of social contact within the care facility ($r = 0.39$, $p < .05$); satisfaction with religion correlated positively with the frequency of religious practice ($r = 0.46$, $p < .05$) and satisfaction with health was negatively correlated with illness in the past year ($r = -0.49$, $p < .01$).

The relationship between general life satisfaction and the domain-specific indicators, both objective and subjective, was also carried out. In contrast to the baseline findings, only four of the subjective life domain scores were found to correlate with general life satisfaction; satisfaction ratings of finances, religion, health and safety were found to be positively correlated with satisfaction with life in general.

Only two of the domain-specific objective indicators were found to be correlated with general life satisfaction. Objective indices of living situation were found to be correlated positively with general life satisfaction suggesting that the physical comfort, privacy and sense of belonging in the home or care facility were related to clients' general sense of well-being. Illness in the past year was found to be negatively correlated with global quality of life. It is interesting to note that indices of health, both objective and subjective, emerge as important influences of general life satisfaction for this group of clients. This is not altogether surprising as health is likely to be an important consideration for this client group many of whom are quite elderly.

Relationship of quality of life indices to the other outcome measures

As the move to the community resulted in a number of significant improvements in behavioural functioning (see chapter 4 it was important to monitor the effect of these changes on clients' quality of life. The relationship of general quality of life to overall levels of dependency and psychiatric functioning was examined (see Table 6.3). At twelve months post-discharge, no significant relationship was found between general life satisfaction and overall levels of dependency as measured by the Total General Behaviour score on the REHAB scale. The relationship at hospital baseline indicated that increased levels of satisfaction were associated with higher levels of dependency, however, for the sub-group of discharged clients, overall levels of social and behavioural functioning do not appear to be related to general life satisfaction in the community.

The relationship of general quality of life to levels of psychiatric functioning at twelve months post-discharge was also examined. As may be seen in Table 6.3, no significant relationships were found between general life satisfaction and either overall levels of psychopathology as measured by the total BPRS score, or selected individual item scores. The correlations between general life satisfaction and the indices of psychopathology were examined over the course of the study and it was found that the pattern does not remain stable across the pre-discharge and post-discharge points. While levels of depression and thought disorder were found to be related to general life satisfaction across the hospital phase of the study, at six and twelve months post-discharge this relationship is not maintained. In general, the influence of levels of psychiatric symptomatology on general quality of life appears to alter following discharge from hospital, taking on less significance. Although one would be cautious about drawing conclusions from a relatively small sample, it does seem to suggest that the nature of the relationship is not a stable one and that quality of life in the community for this group of clients may be influenced more significantly by factors other than psychiatric state. It would be interesting to ascertain if this pattern would be replicated with a larger sample size.

The pattern of change in quality of life indices

Of particular interest was the pattern of change in the quality of life measures over the course of the study taking into account the three pre-discharge hospital assessments and the three post-discharge community assessments. A retrospective analysis across the baseline and community

156

data points was carried out for the discharged group separately. As may been from the analysis of the post-discharge data the impact of the move to the community on clients' quality of life can be most clearly observed in relation to the objective life domain indices. Significant changes were found in relation to the living objective scale ($F = 4.48$, $p < .01$), the social objective scale ($F = 8.41$, $p < .001$), and the leisure objective scale ($F = 3.50$, $p < .01$). The nature of the changes in the living situation, social relations and leisure activities have already been discussed and are clearly attributable to the change in living style following the move to the community. The validity of these findings is supported by the other measures being used in the study which also point to improved care environments, more client oriented care practices and increased levels of social and behavioural functioning (see Crosby et al., this volume; Crosby, Barry, Carter and Lowe, 1993). However, not all of these changes are mirrored in the subjective measures. Given the discrepancy between the subjective and objective indices it was of particular interest to monitor the degree of fluctuation in the subjective measures of life satisfaction across the course of the study for the discharged group.

Repeated measures analyses of variance (MANOVA) were carried out on the subjective composite indices across the six data collection points for the group of hospital leavers. The only subjective scale to show any significant change across the course of the study was the satisfaction with living situation scale ($F = 3.12$, $p < .01$). This finding is in keeping with the results from the comparison of the post-discharge scores with the hospital baseline. Levels of satisfaction in relation to the living situation scale are depicted in Figure 6.3, as expected the increases in satisfaction coincide with the move from hospital and remain relatively stable across the three post-discharge points. None of the other subjective indices show any significant changes following the move to the community. It is also interesting in this respect, to look at levels of general satisfaction across the six data points. As Figure 6.4 depicts, levels of general life satisfaction show an initial increase just after the move to the community placements and this change was found to be significantly higher than baseline levels at both the six weeks and six months post-discharge points. However, at twelve months post-discharge the satisfaction levels appear to settle back to their pre-discharge levels, but still remaining relatively high. Overall, however, the pattern of change in general life satisfaction across pre and post-discharge points is not statistically significant. These findings suggest that the subjective indices are relatively stable and are not merely a function of mood or other transient influences at the time of judgement as suggested by researchers such as Strack, Schwarz, Chassein, Kern and Wagner (1990) and Schwarz and Strack (1990).

157

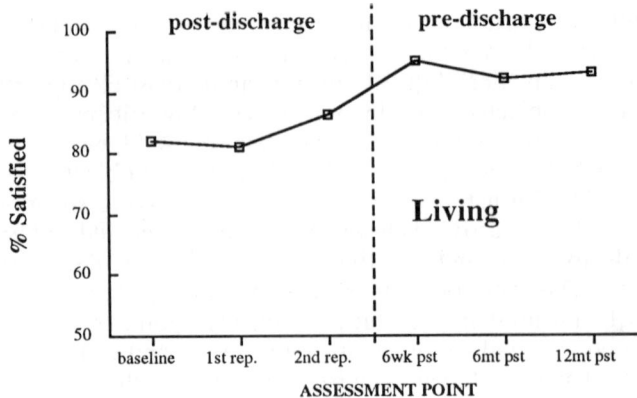

Figure 6.3
Levels of satisfaction with living situation across pre and post-discharge assessment points

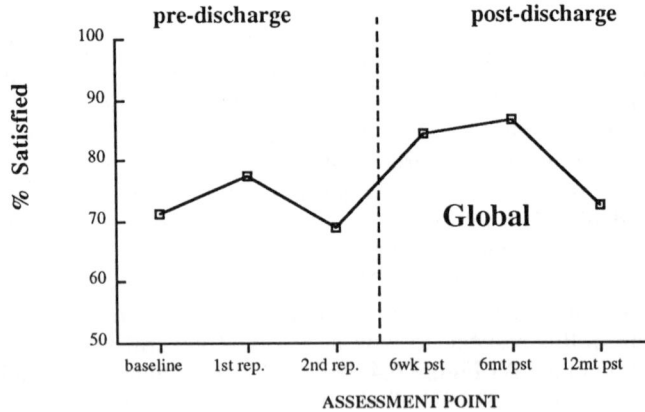

Figure 6.4
Levels of general life satisfaction across pre and post-discharge assessment points

However, the relative stability of the satisfaction ratings across the hospital and community phases of the study does raise some concern in relation to the sensitivity of these measures in tapping changes in external life conditions. The adequacy of satisfaction ratings in reflecting levels of subjective well-being would still appear to be in doubt. This point will be returned to in the discussion section.

Discussion

The results of the quality of life study support the findings from previous research which suggests that people with chronic psychiatric disabilities can live in the community successfully (Dickey, Gudeman, Hellman, Donatelle and Grinspoon, 1981; Stein and Test, 1978; Okin et al. 1983) and that given the right environment and adequate resources, chronic dependent clients do have the capacity for developing an improved quality of life (Murphy, 1991). For the present sample, the majority of whom were discharged into supported residential settings, the movement to the community resulted in improvements in objective standards of living, higher levels of interactive contact within the facility, increased leisure activity and greater personal freedom and independence. The majority have adapted well to their life in the community and clearly express a preference for community living over life in hospital. This adjustment is worthy of comment given the relatively lengthy periods this group had spent in hospital.

The reported increase in social interaction within the community facilities is consistent with the findings from other studies of people moved from large institutions to smaller domestic units (Gibbons and Butler, 1989; Garety and Morris, 1984). However, at this stage it is difficult to assess the actual level of integration and acceptance in the local community as clients' social network is mainly restricted to contact with other clients and staff in the resettlement programme. As may be seen from the results, significant changes were not found in all life areas e.g. family contact and finance remain common sources of dissatisfaction. This finding is consistent with that reported by previous studies (Baker and Intagliata 1982; Lehman et al., 1986). It is likely, however, as pointed out by Petch (1990) and Okin et al. (1983), that change in the more long-term patterns of behaviour will probably take longer to be attained.

As measured by the quality of life indices, the most significant changes are in relation to the immediate living situation with improvements in living conditions reflected in significant increases in satisfaction with living conditions. This finding is in keeping with that reported by Lehman et al. (1986) in their comparison of the quality of life of clients in hospital and community residences. Shadish et al. (1985) have also pointed to the importance of the quality of the immediate environment as a predictor of self-reports of well-being. These results are encouraging with respect to the impact of more 'normalised' living conditions on clients' quality of life. The increase in the sense of freedom and independence reported by individual clients is clearly linked to the more 'normalised' care environments and the more client-oriented care process brought about as a result of the move from hospital. The more 'personalised' living environments have facilitated a greater sense of belonging than in the hospital and the high degree of community accessibility has led to more participation in the local community through activities such as shopping, going to the pub, and attending evening classes. Clients highly value their greater independence, even in small matters such as 'choosing my own food' or doing their own shopping. Clients also pointed to the importance of being treated with 'decency and respect', which suggests that the attitude as well as the working practices of care staff may indeed by a crucial determinant of quality of life for clients in residential care either in hospital or in the community. The care staff in the community schemes were found to generally have very positive attitudes concerning their work and showed high levels of commitment and interest in the clients' welfare (see chapter 3). This situation contrasts with the low morale of many hospital staff and the depersonalisation that many clients experience in the environment of the large hospital. The reported improvements in quality of life would therefore appear to be strongly related to both the changes in the standard of the care environment and in the quality of care provided.

The importance of improved care practices accompanying improved standards of living has been highlighted in a recent study of the quality of life of schizophrenic out-patients by Skantze, Malm, Dencker, May and Corrigan (1992). It was found that once a 'normal' standard of living is achieved i.e. one that approximates to that of the general population, this in itself does not generate a high quality of life. In other words, the study found that there was no correlation between standard of living and subjective quality of life in a chronic population once a minimum standard of living had been reached. While raising the standard of living for discharged clients to that of members of the local community is obviously a very important goal of resettlement programmes, there is also a need to bring about change in the care process with the aim of enhancing and facilitating improved quality of life for clients. In this respect, data from quality of life interviews can give important pointers about how the goal of maximising quality of life may be translated into practice for carers and also the extent to which this aim is being successfully achieved.

Chapter 3 outlines the positive features of the care process in the community care schemes in this study; the reduction in restrictive care practices, the adoption of more client-oriented care management procedures and client involvement in decision-making. These changes in the care process have clearly registered with clients as the major differences between hospital and community care and are reflected in comments concerning the greater independence and freedom afforded by the community settings;

'Independence, choosing my own food, cooking, cleaning, clearing' , 'got more freedom to do what you want to do',
'It's a better type of life altogether, there's freedom and happiness like I never had before.'

Although lack of freedom per se did not emerge in clients' accounts of life in the hospital it would appear that independence and being able to do things for oneself, once experienced, is a very important consideration for chronic clients. Rosenfield (1992) presents a theoretical model which proposes that the critical components of care for the subjective quality of life of chronic psychiatric clients are those aspects of the service which enhance clients' perceptions of perceived control and personal mastery. The findings from the present study would appear to support this model. As may be seen from clients' accounts of their experiences, perceptions of control over their lives was significantly enhanced as a result of the more liberal and empowering care regimes in the community settings; 'I feel I'm in control, I can be my own boss'. It is interesting to note that evidence for this outcome emerges largely from the qualitative data rather than from the life domain indices. It would seem that in future studies of the quality of life of chronic clients it would be useful to assess more directly perceptions of individual autonomy and to include a measure of perceived control. Although implied in some of the life domain scales, the addition of items specifically tapping independence or freedom would increase the content validity of the quality of life interview for a chronic population.

Concerning the sensitivity of the quality of the life indices, the impact of the move to the community on clients' quality of life can be most clearly observed in relation to the objective life domain indices, registering improvements in living conditions, social relations and increased leisure activities. However, the impact of these changes on clients' sense of well-being is not immediately clear from the subjective measures, as there is no overall increase in life satisfaction apart from satisfaction with living situation. The quality of life indices do not indicate the extent to which the improvements in the objective life domain scores are being translated into increased levels of subjective well-being. It is quite clear, however, from clients' statements that the move to the community has had a considerably positive impact on their lives. Clients comment on the changes in their outlook; 'I see the future as good', 'I'm enjoying life like never before', and how they value being 'treated with decency and respect' in the community settings. However, these critical changes are not being tapped by the satisfaction measures which remain relatively stable across both the hospital and the community phases of the study.

As the correlational findings indicate, satisfaction measures do not appear to be strongly related to their objective counterparts. This finding calls into question the sensitivity of the satisfaction measures. Glatzer (1991) reports that individuals may experience feelings of satisfaction and deprivation at the same time, and indeed the findings from the hospital phase of the present study would support this. The occurrence of this disjunction between the objective and subjective components of quality of life points to the need for further exploration of the mediating mechanisms by which these different constituents of quality of life are appraised. The nature of the relationship between objective and subjective indicators is obviously complex and it would appear that there is not a one to one mapping between objective conditions and subjective well-being. It would therefore seem important in the development of quality of life research in this area to now examine the possible mediators of subjective well-being for chronic clients, and to delineate those factors which determine how individuals perceive and judge their quality of life.

Data from the present study suggests that we need to consider issues of personal autonomy and perceived control as being central to the effort of assessing perceived quality of life, as these are clearly of considerable importance to people with chronic mental health problems who are service dependent. Constructs such as autonomy and perceived control emerge as important determinants of subjective well-being for clients in the present study. However, neither of these constructs were measured directly by the life domain indices. Despite the emphasis given to the concept of satisfaction in the quality of life literature, it may be advisable to move from a reliance on satisfaction as the sole dimension along which subjective well-being should be measured. As discussed earlier in relation to the hospital baseline findings, the construct of satisfaction is influenced by a whole host of cognitive and affective factors, many of which directly affect the lives of chronic psychiatric clients; restricted life experiences, low aspirations, limited expectations, atypical social comparison standards as a result of institutional living, and generally a life history hampered by chronic psychiatric problems and high levels of dependency. It would therefore seem essential that we review the constructs that may be important mediators of subjective well-being for chronic clients, looking to concepts such as perceived control and personal autonomy in addition to life satisfaction.

Conclusions

The quality of life outcomes do provide support for the claim that it is possible to maintain even the more dependent, chronic psychiatric clients in the community and increase their quality of life through the provision of carefully designed and adequately supported community residential schemes. Given the lack of correlation between the indices of psychiatric and behavioural functioning and general life satisfaction in the community settings, it would appear that level of functioning alone is not the key determinant of improved quality of life. A study by Champney and Dzurec (1992), reporting that changes in symptomatology and functioning may only have a limited bearing on reports of life satisfaction in chronic psychiatric clients, would tend to support this assertion. In the present study, improvements in the standard of the care environments and the quality of the care provided emerge as the critical determinants in bringing about improved life quality. However, these results must be interpreted with some caution. The period of one year post-discharge is relatively short in terms of the history of contact with the services for many of the clients in the study. It is important that progress over a longer follow-up period should be monitored, perhaps on an annual basis, in order to ensure that standards of care and positive client outcomes are being maintained.

In the lifetime of the study, it was possible to follow up only a small number of clients from the original cohort, and generalisation of the findings to other schemes is of course dependent on the quality of care provision following discharge. Due to the small sample size it was not possible to explore differences in the quality of life offered by different community settings. As the study concentrates mainly on care schemes providing 24 hour support, it cannot comment on the impact of community placement on clients in independent living or family settings, who in many senses may be most at risk of inadequate service provision. There is also a need to look more closely at the standard of care in private care homes as there may be great variability in the quality of care provided. It was not possible to examine these issues in the present study due to the small number of clients discharged into these settings. Another area which remains largely unexplored is the gender and age differences that may exist in the factors which clients perceive as important in their quality of life.

Despite these limitations, the quality of life study does provide evidence that it is possible to measure quality of life in a meaningful way for continuing care clients and therefore allows for potential comparisons with different client groups in different locations. The study demonstrates the utility of quality of life as an evaluative framework against which to assess the outcomes of care, providing a useful tool for incorporating the clients' perspectives into the evaluation process. There is clearly need for further development in the measurement of the concept of quality of life for this client group in order to understand more fully its meaning and its implications for theory and practice. At a theoretical level there is need for greater attention to be directed to the appraisal process involved in self-assessed judgements of quality of life. The types of cognitive judgements that are made and how these are influenced by standards of social comparison, subjective perceptual processes and internal states such as needs, knowledge, beliefs, values and attitudes requires further study. The importance of internal referents such as level of aspiration, comparison level and perceived control as mediators of subjective quality of life experience have been emphasised by Gutek, Allen, Tyler, Lau and Majchrzak (1983). However, the influence of these factors in relation to psychiatric populations has not been explored despite their obvious relevance. It is important that further developments in the measurement of quality of life be informed by a more coherent theoretical model of the process of appraisal and the type of mediating variables which need to be taken into account.

As an outcome measure of care provision, it is important that future evaluation studies should attempt to link the quality of life data to elements of the care process in order to identify those components which are critical for ensuring a good quality of life for clients. In this way the quality of life data may be successfully used to inform the development of care practices and to suggest types of service input which may empower clients and enhance their life quality. These may be areas of work and finance as suggested by Rosenfield (1992) or simply being treated with dignity and respect as suggested by clients in the present study.

References

Andrews, R.F., and Withey, S.B. (1976), *Social indicators of well-being: Americans' perceptions of life quality.* New York: Plenum Press.

Anthony, W.A. (1980), *The principles of psychiatric rehabilitation.* Baltimore: University Park Press.

Bachrach, L.L. (1980), 'Is the least restrictive environment always the best? Sociological and semantic implications', *Hospital and Community Psychiatry,* 31, 97-103.

Baker, F. and Intagliata, J. (1982), 'Quality of life in the evaluation of community support systems', *Evaluation and Program Planning,* 5, 69-79.

Barry, M.M., Crosby, C. and Mitchell, D.A. (1992), 'Quality of life issues in the evaluation of mental health services', in D.R. Trent (ed.), *Promotion of Mental Health,* Vol. 1. (pp. 153-163). Aldershot: Avebury.

Barry, M.M., Crosby, C. and Bogg, J. (1993), 'Methodological issues in evaluating the quality of life of long-stay psychiatric patients', *Journal of Mental Health,* 2, 43-56.

Barry, M.M. and Crosby, C. (1993), 'Community mental health care: Promoting a better quality of life for long-term clients', in D.R. Trent and C. Reed (eds.), *Promotion of Mental Health,* Vol. 2. (pp. 113-130). Aldershot: Avebury.

Barry, M.M. and Crosby, C. (1994), 'Quality of life and mental health: Evaluating the impact of long-term care', in I. Markova and R.M. Farr (eds), *Representations of Health, Illness and Handicap.* Harwood Academic Press. (in press)

Bartlett, D.P. and Intagliata, J. (1985), *A value-relative assessment of the quality of life of chronic psychiatric patients.* Unpublished manuscript.

Bigelow, D.A., Brodsky, G., Stewart, L. and Olson, M. (1982), 'The concept and measurement of quality of life as a dependent variable in evaluation of mental health services', in G.J. Tash and W.R. Tash (eds.), *Innovative Approaches to Mental Health Evaluation* (pp. 345-366). New York: Academic Press.

Campbell, A., Converse, P.E., and Rodgers, W.L. (1976), *The quality of American life*. New York: Russell Sage Foundation.

Carstenson, L.L. and Cone, J.D. (1983), 'Social desirability and the measurement of psychological well-being in elderly persons', *Journal of Gerontology*, 38, 713-715.

Champney, T.F. and Dzurec, L.C. (1992), 'Involvement in productive activities and satisfaction with living situation among severely mentally disabled adults', *Hospital and Community Psychiatry*, 43, 9, 899-903.

Coid, J.W. (1993), 'Quality of life for patients detained in hospital', *British Journal of Psychiatry*, 162, 611-620.

Crosby, C., Barry, M.M., Mitchell, D.A., Grant, P., Horrocks, F.A., and Littlejohns, C.S. (1990), *Evaluation of the Clwyd mental health community service: An interim report*. Health Services Research Unit, Department of Psychology, University College of North Wales: Unpublished Manuscript.

Crosby, C. and Barry, M.M. (1991), *Community care - initial findings - 6 weeks after discharge from North Wales Hospital*. Health Services Research Unit, Department of Psychology, University College of North Wales: Unpublished Manuscript.

Crosby, C., Barry, M.M., Carter, M.F. and Lowe, C.F. (1993), 'Psychiatric rehabilitation and community care: Resettlement from North Wales Hospital', *Health and Social Care*, 1, 355-363.

Dickey, B., Gudeman, J., Hellman, S. Donatelle, A., Grinspoon, L. (1981), 'A follow-up study of deinstitutionalized chronic patients four years after discharge', *Hospital and Community Psychiatry*, 32, 326-330.

Garety, P.A. and Morris, I. (1984), 'A new unit for long-stay psychiatric patients: Organisation, attitudes and quality of life', *Psychological Medicine*, 14, 183-192.

Gibbons, J.S. and Butler, J.P. (1987), 'Quality of life for 'new' long-stay psychiatric in-patients: The effects of moving to a hostel', *British Journal of Psychiatry*, 157, 347-354.

Glatzer, W. (1991), 'Quality of life in advanced industrialised countries: the case of West Germany', in F. Strack, M. Argyle and N. Schwarz (eds.), *Subjective Well-Being* (pp. 261-279). Oxford: Pergammon.

Gutek, B.A., Allen, H., Tyler, T.R., Lau, R.R. and Majchrzak, A. (1983), 'The importance of internal referents as determinants of satisfaction', *Journal of Community Psychology*, 11, 111-120.

Jones, K., Robinson, M. and Golightley, M. (1986), 'Long-term psychiatric patients in the community', *British Journal of Psychiatry*, 149, 537-540.

Hall, J.N. and Baker, R. (1983), *REHAB*. Aberdeen: Vine Publishing Company.

Lehman, A.F., Ward, N.C., and Linn, L.S. (1982), 'Chronic mental patients: The quality of life issue', *American Journal of Psychiatry*, 139, 1271-1276.

Lehman, A.F. (1983a), 'The well-being of chronic mental patients: Assessing their quality of life', *Archives of General Psychiatry*, 40, 369-373.

Lehman, A.F. (1983b), 'The effects of psychiatric symptoms on quality of life assessments among the chronically mentally ill', *Evaluation and Program Planning*, 6, 143-151.

Lehman, A.F., Possidente, S. and Hawker, F. (1986), 'The quality of life of chronic patients in a state hospital and in community residences', *Hospital and Community Psychiatry*, 37, 901-907.

Lehman, A.F. (1988), 'A quality of life interview for the chronically mentally ill', *Evaluation and Program Planning*, 11, 51-62.

Murphy, E. (1991), *After the asylums: Community care for people with mental illness*. London: Faber and Faber.

Okin, R.L., Dolnick, J.A. and Pearsall, D.T. (1983), 'Patients' perspectives on community alternatives to hospitalisation: A follow-up study', *American Journal of Psychiatry*, 140, 1460-1464.

Overall, J. and Gorham, D. (1962), 'The Brief Psychiatric Rating Scale', *Psychological Reports*, 10, 799-812.

Perkins, R.E., Hollyman, J.A., Boardman, C.J., Humphreys-Hunt, B., Reeves, C., and Weizmann, E. (1992), 'From long-stay patient to Sloane Ranger: Outcome of resettlement of 15 old-long-stay psychiatric patients in 'warden supervised' accommodation for the elderly', *Journal of Mental Health*, 1, 149-162.

Petch, A. (1990), *'Heaven Compared to a Hospital Ward': An evaluation of eleven supported accommodation projects for those with mental health problems*. Social Work Research Centre, Stirling University.

Pinkey, A.A., Gerber, G.J., Lafave, H.G. (1991), 'Quality of life after psychiatric rehabilitation: the clients' perspective', *Acta Psychiatric Scandinavica*, 83, 86-91.

Rosenfield, S. (1992), 'Factors contributing to the subjective quality of life of the chronic mentally ill', *Journal of Health and Social Behaviour*, 33, 4, 299-315.

Sartorius, N. (1992), 'Rehabilitation and quality of life', *Hospital and Community Psychiatry*, 43, 12, 1180-1181.

Schwarz, N. and Strack, F. (1990), 'Evaluating one's life: A judgement model of subjective well-being', In F. Strack, M. Argyle and N. Schwarz (eds.) *Subjective Well-Being* (pp. 27-47). Oxford: Pergammon.

Shadish, W.R., Orwin, R.G., Silber, B.G. and Bootzin, R.R. (1985), 'The subjective well-being of mental patients in nursing homes', *Evaluation and Program Planning*, 8, 239-250.

Simpson, C.J., Hyde, C.E. and Farragher, E.B. (1989), 'The chronically mentally ill in community facilities: A study of quality of life', *British Journal of Psychiatry*, 154, 77-82.

Skantze, K., Malm, U., Dencker, S.J., May, P.R.A., Corrigan, P. (1992), 'Comparison of quality of life with standard of living in schizophrenic out-patients', *British Journal of Psychiatry,* 161, 797-801.

Strack, F., Schwarz, N., Chassein, B., Kern, D. and Wagner, D. (1990), 'Salience of comparison standards and the activation of social norms: Consequences for judgements of happiness and their communication', *British Journal of Social Psychology*, 29, 303-314.

Stein, L.I. and Test, M.A. (eds), (1978), *Alternatives to mental hospital treatment.* New York: Plenum.

Ware, J. (1978), 'Effects of acquiescent response set on patient satisfaction ratings', *Medical Care*, 16, 327-336.

Wilde, E.D. and Svanberg, P.O. (1990), 'Never mind the width - measure the quality', *Clinical Psychology Forum*, 2-5.

7 Costing hospital and community care for long-stay psychiatric patients

Neil Garrod and Sandra Vick

Summary

Mental health service provision in the community is quite different to that offered in traditional hospital type institutions. This chapter offers insights into the comparative economic consequences of the two types of care. It further highlights the significant differences in costings for different forms of community care schemes.

An innovative aspect of this work is the identification of institutional decisions as significant in the eventual level of costing for different care forms. It becomes clear from the results of this study that care can be as cheap or expensive as the policy makers wish. In the absence of a clear, needs based assessment measure to guide care provision, a change from large institution to community care will not, of itself, influence the cost of such care provision. What it does do is offer policy makers the opportunity to reconsider the nature and quality of care provided and thus improve the quality of life of long stay psychiatric clients.

Introduction

Costing healthcare provision

An integral part of the North Wales study was a comprehensive costing exercise. The aim of this section of the study was to identify the resources used in hospital care and the various community care settings; to measure the costs of those resources; to compare the costs of hospital-based with community based care; to determine the costs falling to different agencies; and to identify factors which might be driving care costs. This is considered an important aspect of the study as the government's document

'Care in the Community' has led to 'a general and growing groundswell of opinion which is questioning the way in which so-called community care policies are operating in practice' (DHSS, 1985). Community care is seen as a cheap alternative, releasing the government from any responsibility of care provision for the mentally ill (Herman and Green, 1991).

In a world of limited resources allocations cannot be based purely on clinical judgments or the views of service planners but on a carefully designed economic evaluation of the different alternatives. Economics, as defined by Samuelson (1976) is;'

> The study of how men and society end up choosing, with or without the use of money, to employ scarce productive resources that could have alternative uses, to produce various commodities and distribute them for consumption, now or in the future, among various people and groups in society. It analyses the costs and benefits of improving patterns of resource allocation.

Hence an economic evaluation incorporates the measurement of both costs and benefits of using scarce resources, such as funding for mental health care. The aim of an economic evaluation is to alleviate concerns of 'cost-cutting', to answer the questions regarding 'value for money', and to provide evidence about economic efficiency in the allocation of resources.

Economic evaluation techniques

The trend towards the use of economic evaluation in multi-disciplinary analysis has brought with it new appraisal techniques. Among these, two in particular have been used in costing social care: cost benefit analysis (CBA) and cost effectiveness analysis (CEA).

A cost benefit analysis evaluation compares alternative policies, according to a comparison of costs and benefits, measured in purely monetary terms. Since each alternative is assessed in monetary values, it can be examined on its own merits. Writers such as Alan Williams (1974) discuss how cost benefit analysis can be used to aid decision making with regards to health service policy and Klarman (1974) considers its utilisation in assessing technology in health services, while Weisbrod, Test and Stein (1980) discuss the determination of the benefits and costs of alternatives to mental hospital treatment. A fuller description of cost benefit analysis can be found in Bohm (1987).

One of the main difficulties in implementing cost benefit analysis in costing social care is the problem of placing pecuniary values on all of the costs and benefits of particular alternatives. In the private sector, a firm has prices for total input and output, and is able to determine the costs of production with relative ease. In the social care setting, goods are 'zero-priced' at the point of consumption and, therefore, do not provide easy access to the costs of services. In order to determine the cost of providing a service in a particular unit, transfer pricing is used. This involves allocating costs to an unit according to its use of resources. This is purely a paper transfer, which enables the determination of some of the costs involved, but not all.

Weisbrod and Helming (1980) identify several drawbacks to the use of cost benefit analysis in the field of psychiatry. They claim they were 'unable to obtain any data on the burdens that mental patients impose on neighbours, co-workers and others outside their families' and were 'unable to provide monetary values for a number of forms of costs and benefits' for which they had developed quantitative measures (p. 616). In an attempt to overcome these difficulties cost effectiveness analysis was developed. In this approach monetary costs of alternatives are evaluated with respect to the non monetary outcomes which they produce. A comparison of monetary costs and benefits, and non monetary outcomes is then undertaken.

The need for both cost and quality questions to be answered has led to a growing use of cost-effectiveness analysis in evaluating the provision of mental health care world wide. In the USA, Pennhurst Mental Retardation Centre was put under a court order to deinstitutionalise its clients, and move them into community settings. A study by Conroy and Bradley (1985) looked at the monetary and social effects of this court order. A unit cost examination of the Pennhurst Mental Retardation Centre programmes, compared to those programmes in operation in community situations, uncovered variations in costs across the programmes. Regression analysis was used to identify the reasons for these cost differences. Overall, community care was found to be the cheapest cost option due to a number of influencing variables, including time spent with clients (47.6%), type of facility (10.2%), programme size (11.9%), and year of operation (13.8%). Conroy and Bradley, also suggest that, 'to some extent clients are fitted to programme models, as much, if not more than programme models are fit to clients'. The use of regression analysis, and the question of care type cost impact, are both critical questions which recur in most studies and which will be examined in more detail in due course.

In West Germany, Hafner and an der Heiden (1989a) evaluated the cost-effectiveness of caring for schizophrenic patients in the community. The mean cost of care in the community was found to be less than half that of the traditional hospital care, but 6% of the cohort in the study received care that was more costly than that of traditional care. Hafner and an der Heiden also discovered it to be considerably cheaper if severely ill and disabled patients needing particularly intensive care are not discharged from the hospital. The authors conclude that community care has a slight overall economic advantage over hospital care and no clear disadvantage in treatment results.

In Italy, the government funded the movement of clients into the community from hospitals. Tansella (1991) found improvement in the psychiatric condition of clients in community care compared to hospital care. As yet the results from the accompanying research into costs of care have not been published.

In England and Wales, the research involving the use of cost-effectiveness analysis in mental health evaluations, has been in both mental handicap and mental health. There is no work published as yet on evaluations in Scotland, as it has a different policy for mental health care. There are six main studies involving cost-effectiveness analysis in mental health evaluations: three concern the transfer of psychiatric clients from institutions to community based care and three, the similar transfer of individuals with mental handicap.

Martin Knapp and Jenny Beecham have been involved in two major studies concerning the cost of community mental health care in England. Knapp and Beecham (1990a), as part of the TAPS project have undertaken a study of the gradual transfer of psychiatric patients from Friern and Claybury hospitals into community care. They produced costs suggesting that community care can be less expensive even when the whole range of economic costs are taken into account. Knapp and Beecham (1990a and 1990b) have used similar methodology for an analysis undertaken for the DHSS. The DHSS (1983) needed the study 'to demonstrate methods that are both beneficial to the people concerned and cost effective'. Knapp and Beecham collected information on the cost of care provision for some 900 people in mental hospitals around Britain. With follow-up investigations, they found few negative outcomes from moves into the community by the previous hospital residents. From the results of their study, they show community care to be less expensive and more beneficial than in-patient hospital care. Regression analysis is used to examine the extent to which the costs of community care can be explained by client baseline characteristics. Those clients with fewer behavioural problems and symptoms receive relatively less expensive care packages than those with higher levels of dependency.

A comparison between Maudsley and Bethlem Royal Hospital (a postgraduate teaching hospital), the psychiatric wing of St. Francis Hospital and Cane Hill (a large psychiatric hospital) is undertaken by Wykes (1982). As far as revenue costs are concerned, the components due to nursing staff are similar in Maudsley and Bethlem and St. Francis, but are three times as high as those for Cane Hill. She found that one of the reasons for the costs of mental hospital care for elderly, long stay residents being so low is that the service is under staffed. Wykes concludes that transfer to a large mental hospital of such patients would be cheaper but at the expense of a lower quality of life and a lower standard of care due to a lower staff-patient ratio.

Most studies investigating the transfer of mentally handicapped clients from large institutions into community care have found that community care is in fact more expensive than hospital care. Wright and Haycox (1985) comparing the costs of small scale facilities for the mentally handicapped with those of a long stay hospital found that the former facilities are more expensive. Davies (1987) compares the costs and quality of different residential services for people with mental handicap. The major resource used by all services evaluated is staff time. Staff costs account for 80% of total costs in the results of the study, and are seen to be a major influence on the higher costs in the community settings.

Over the last thirty years the transfer of clients from hospital to community care has not been very rapid, therefore very few studies have been able to investigate the cost-effective analysis of the complete closure of a hospital. Korman and Glennerster (1990) follow the closure of Darenth hospital, and are thus able to provide an insight into the full benefits of available community versus hospital care and discovered wide ranges in the annual costs of facilities. Small group houses have higher costs than more institutionalised forms of residential care. Overall, community type care for mentally handicapped individuals is more costly than the old large Victorian hospital, but it is far easier to staff the community homes than it had been in the hospital. Their conclusion is 'more humane care costs more' (p. 157, Korman and Glennerster, 1990).

Cost collection in North Wales Hospital

The resources costed in this study are outlined in Table 7.1 and are similar to those used in studies by Wright et al. (1981) and Korman and Glennester (1990). The costs were collected on an average basis as in studies by May (1971), Conroy and Bradley (1985), and Glennester (1990). The study attempts to cost care provision in existing institutional care settings and compare them with the costs of caring for the same clients in various community care settings.

Costs are collected for resources used by the cohort of 63 individuals living in four different wards in North Wales Hospital (NWH) (see chapter 2 for a detailed description of the characteristics of the sample). These costs are compared across the four wards, and are used to determine factors influencing costs, in order to identify possible cost structures in community settings. The 63 individuals were awaiting transfer into care settings in the neighbouring community. NWH houses Ward 2, 3 and 4 and an annex houses Ward 1. Ward 1 had a closure programme scheduled for November 1990, and therefore, the provision of service was being run down, as were resident numbers (from over 100 to 26 by October 1990).

A simple statistical study of the baseline characteristics of the individuals in the four wards was undertaken (Table 7.2). Knapp & Beecham (1989) found that men cost £20 more a week to care for than do women in the community. The four wards in the present study are predominantly male, with only 8 females out of 63 patients. This could have important implications for community/hospital cost comparisons.

Terms. As described in chapter 2 the data indicate two groups of patients. Patients in Wards 1 and 2 may be described as old long-stay patients (OLSP) as they exhibit older age, longer average duration of stay per admission, longer length of stay, and higher total years of hospitalisation. Patients in Wards 3 and 4, may be described as the new long-stay patients (NSLP) as they are younger, have shorter duration of stay per admission, have shorter length of stay and less total years of hospitalisation.

Table 7.1
Outline of main cost categories

Resources	Including:	Valuation Method	Price Basis
A] Care Staff Services	Nurses and care salaries	Salaries, including night/ weekend rates, including employers contributions	Ward 1989/90 Home 1990/91
B] External Services	Consultant Psychiarist S.H.O./Junior Officer Community Psychiatric Nurse (CPN), G.P., Dentist, Social Worker Day Care, Occupational Therapist.	Proportion of salary time spent on ward/in home divided between the no. of residents. Cost per attendance.	Ward 1989/90 Home 1990/91
C] General Services	General Hospital Overheads, Eg., Domestic Staff, Energy Laundry Service, Estate Management. Day-to-day Home Expenses Community Charge, Admin. Staff Training course expenses & Travel expenses claimed. .	Total cost to hospital/ home divided equally between the residents.	Ward 1989/90 Home 1990/91
D] Personal Comsumption	Pocket money from DSS and therapeutic earnings.	Individually calculated - average of ward/home.	Ward 1989/90 Home 1990/91
E] EAC of Capital/Rent	EAC of present opportunity costs of buildings, rent charged by housing association	Market Value of Housing with a 60 year life and 5% discount rate.	Ward 1989/90 Home 1990/91

The OLSP have become more institutionalised and less able to look after themselves than the NLSP who show more potential for discharge (see chapter 3).

As rated on the REHAB scale the clients in Ward 1 fall in the 'doubtful if patient could live outside' category, while the residents of the other three wards fall in the 'could live out if supervised' category. The average Total General Behaviour (TGB) scores on the REHAB scale for clients on the 4 wards suggests that clients 'could only live out with much tolerance and supervision'. These scores facilitate estimations of the appropriate care

174

from service requirements of clients. As well as psychiatric symptoms, the patients were rated in terms of physical health. There were no major illnesses or particular disabilities identified on any of the wards nor significant differences between patients on the different wards which might impact on the cost of care provision.

Table 7.2
Baseline characteristics of residents on wards 1-4

Ward			1	2	3	4
Sample			26	10	15	11
Age	-	Mean	68.0	61.2	44.8	39.5
	-	S.D.	7.6	10.0	13.3	11.0
	-	Range	52-87	44-76	27-71	27-64
Sex	-	Males	23	10	15	6
	-	Females	3	0	0	5
Length of stay	-	Mean	32.5	28.8	11.0	3.2
	-	S.D.	14.2	13.6	10.3	2.8
	-	Range	8-62	5-47	0.8-30	0.4-8
Total Years	-	Mean	36.4	33.1	15.2	6.6
Hospitalised	-	S.D.	10.1	8.8	11.6	10.0
	-	Range	19-61	18-45	2-36	1-35
Number of	-	Mean	2	3	5	7
Admissions	-	Range	1-7	1-9	1-16	1-16
Average Duration	-	Mean	27.6	24.1	7.2	1.6
of Stay per	-	S.D.	17.3	15.6	6.4	2.4
Admission yrs.	-	Range	4-61	4-45	0.2-18	0.1-7

Health Authorities produce a set of accounts showing the resource allocation of each hospital in its area, called FR11s. A FR11 is produced for North Wales Hospital (housing Ward 2, Ward 3 and Ward 4) and Ward 1 (as it is a self contained annex). These accounts provide general information regarding resources used in the hospital. In order to gain more ward specific information, interviews were held with charge nurses on the wards. A questionnaire (Garrod and Vick, 1992) is used to guide the interview and provide the necessary information for ward specific resource utilisation. From this information an average cost per patient per ward was generated.

The data were collected for the financial year ending 31 March 1990. Staff costs, external services and personal consumption were calculated from information gained by the questionnaire, with additional information from management accounts in NWH regarding details of employers' contributions and such like. General services resource use was worked out as a hospital average from the FR11s. Capital costs are equivalent annual costs calculated from a buildings valuation by the estate valuers.

The distribution of resource utilisation was similar across the four wards. Table 7.3 shows how the total costs are made up. The largest contributors to total care cost is care staff services and general services.

Table 7.3
Percentage make-up of total ward costs

	Ward 1		Ward 2		Ward 3		Ward 4	
	£	%	£	%	£	%	£	%
Care Staff Services	151.61	47.31	235.95	50.53	212.38	56.62	292.12	62.00
External Services	8.40	2.62	9.37	2.61	24.21	5.59	32.90	6.05
General Services	133.79	41.75	142.41	39.65	137.62	31.80	151.44	27.85
Personal Consumption	12.99	4.05	19.44	5.41	19.40	4.48	15.75	2.90
Capital Costs	13.67	4.27	6.49	1.81	6.49	1.50	6.49	1.19
Total Cost	320.46	100.00	413.66	100.00	400.10	100.00	498.70	100.00

Care staff services are classified as the amount of nursing resources utilised by the clients. Care staff provide the largest cost input into the wards (Table 7.3). This large proportion of staff resource input for providing care for psychiatric patients is found in other studies, eg., Davies (1987), Conroy and Bradley (1985).

Discussions with the charge nurses on the wards revealed that staffing levels have not changed over the last few years and that although patient numbers are not at their maximum, staffing levels have remained the same. Staffing costs can therefore, be seen as a fixed cost. This explains some of the differences in cost of care across the wards. Higher occupancy levels will reduce the average cost per person. Other factors influencing cost are staff qualifications and patient:staff ratios.

In order to produce informative cost of care figures it is important to differentiate between those costs driven by patient need and those which are institutionally based. Occupancy levels, staff qualifications and patient: staff ratios could clearly be influenced by both. In an attempt to identify the primary focus of this study, the needs driven costs, a series of sensitivity analyses were carried out. Whilst these will not identify institutionally driven costs they will expose the potential impact of such factors.

Cost estimates in this study (and all others referenced) are taken at a discrete point in time and so will be influenced by the occupancy and staffing levels at the time of the costings. What needs to be identified is the potential impact on absolute and relative cost estimates of the extant staffing and occupancy levels. For example, is Ward 4 always the most expensive ward over the full range of operationally permissible staffing and occupancy levels? If so we can feel more secure that our costing figures are fully reflective of patient needs. If not, then there is clear evidence that institutional policy decisions are having a significant biasing effect on our cost estimates and they should, therefore, be treated with caution in any cost effectiveness comparison.

Cost sensitivity analyses

The first sensitivity analysis investigated the impact of occupancy level on average patient costs. Three occupancy rates were used; NORM, FULL and NOW. The normal occupancy rate used by the health authority management accounts is 70% of full capacity and is adopted as a 'norm' for each ward [NORM]. The other occupancy rates used in the sensitivity analysis are the full complement [FULL] (this applies to Wards 2, 3 and 4), and the population for each ward at time of collection of costs [NOW]. The sensitivity analysis does not include Ward 1 as there is no available 100% occupancy rate and staff are not fixed due to rapid closure of the ward.

Table 7.4
Cost of care at various occupancy levels

	Full (n=18) 100% occ. level	Now (n=10)	Norm (n=13) 70% occ. level
Ward 2	£	£	£
Care Staff Services	131.09	235.95	181.50
External Services`	9.37	9.37	9.37
General Services	142.41	142.41	142.41
Personal Consumption	19.44	19.44	19.44
Capital Costs	6.49	6.49	6.49
Total Cost	308.80	413.66	359.21
Ward 3	Full (n=18)	Now (n=15)	Norm (n=13)
	£	£	£
Care Staff Services	176.98	212.38	245.05
External Services	24.21	24.21	24.21
General Services	137.62	137.62	137.62
Personal Consumption	19.40	19.40	19.40
Capital Costs	6.49	6.49	6.49
Total Cost	364.70	400.10	432.77
Ward 4	Full(n=18)	Now(n=11)	Norm (n=13)
	£	£	£
Care Staff Services	178.52	292.12	247.18
External Services	32.90	32.90	32.90
General Services	151.44	151.44	151.44
Personal Consumption	15.75	15.75	15.75
Capital Costs	6.49	6.49	6.49
Total Cost	385.10	498.70	453.76

From Table 7.4 it can be seen that Ward 2 had 18 beds and at the time of data collection only 10 were full, a 55% occupancy level. A change of 45% in occupancy level (from NOW to FULL), brings about a fall of 25% in average total cost of care. The costs are spread from £413.66 (NOW) to £308.80 (FULL), giving a range of £104.86 p.w. per resident, 25% of current occupancy costs. The mean cost of care in this range is £360.56.

An occupancy level of 70% produces average total cost per patient per week of £359.21.Whilst it is clear from the results that occupancy has a significant impact on the average cost of care they also provide support for use of the 70% occupancy figure as a 'representative average'. For two out of the three wards the 70% figure is very close to the sensitivity mean value and in the third case the discrepancy is due to currently high occupancy rate which the Health Authority does not expect to continue.

By adopting a common occupancy level across wards the impact of this variable is removed from the cost figures. However, significant differences in care staff costs between wards still exist. Those patients with the highest REHAB Total General Behaviour (TGB) scores (and therefore higher dependency) in Ward 1 and Ward 2 are cheaper to care for than those with lower REHAB TGB scores in Wards 3 and 4.

Another influence on the cost of care is care staff structure. This varies across wards (Table 7.5). Each ward has nurses of various grades; grade I is the most qualified nurse, and grade A is the nursing auxiliary. The wards also have a supply of student nurses at approximately 4.2 students per ward, costed at the midpoint of student scales.

Table 7.5
Grades of staff on each ward

	Day Staff	Night Staff
Ward 1	G,F,3.5E,6B	2E,2A
Ward 2	G,F,2D,0.5B,1/3I	E,D
Ward 3	G,2F,2E,D,2B,1/3I	D,2A
Ward 4	G,4E,3D,1/3I	D,2A,ROTA

The question of optimum mix of staff and the possibilities of employing less qualified staff to do the same job are raised in Mangen et al. (1983). They look at the effect of replacing psychiatric consultants with community psychiatric nurses (CPN). They found that the CPNs were able to keep a much more regular input and be more in touch with the client than the consultants. In order to measure the impact of staff grading in NWH, another sensitivity analysis was undertaken, using four different staff mixes. The mixes chosen were [i] the present mix of nurses, [ii] one high grade nurse (grade G) on the ward supported by the lowest grade (grade A) nurses, [iii] one nurse of each grade, [iv] one high grade, grade G, supported by E grade nurses. The three occupancy rates used above were also introduced into the analysis to investigate the combined influence of occupancy rate and staff mix. The sensitivity analysis produces a matrix of total costs at different staff mixes and occupancy rates as displayed in Tables 7.6, 7.7 and 7.8.

Table 7.6
The effect on the total cost of care of variations in care staff grade mixes and occupancy levels (%) on ward 2

	Number of residents on the ward		
	n=18 100% £	n=10 55% £	n=13 70% £
Staff mix			
[i] 0.33I,G,F,2D,0.5B.	308.80	413.66	359.21
[ii] 0.33I,G,3.5A.	293.57	386.26	338.13
[iii] 0.33I,G,F,E,D,0.5C.	310.44	416.61	361.48
[iv] 0.33I,G,3.5E.	312.33	420.03	364.11

Table 7.7
The effect on the total cost of care of variations in care staff grade mixes and occupancy levels (%) on ward 3

	Number of residents in ward		
	n=18 100% £	n=15 83% £	n=13 70% £
[i] 0.33I,G,2F,2E,D,2B	364.70	400.10	432.77
[ii] 0.33I,G,7A	333.64	362.82	389.76
[iii] 0.33I,G,F,E,D,C,B,3A.	352.43	385.37	415.78
[iv] 0.33I,G,7E.	371.15	407.84	441.71

Table 7.8
The effect on the total cost of care of variations in care staff grade mixes and occupancy levels (%) on ward 4

	Number of residents in ward 3		
	n=18 100% £	n=11 61% £	n=13 70% £
Staff Mix			
[i] 0.33I,G,4E,3D	385.10	498.70	453.76
[ii] 0.33I,G,7A	360.47	458.39	419.66
[iii] 0.33I,G,F,E,D,C,B,2A	380.33	490.89	447.15
[iv] 0.33I,G,7E	397.98	519.78	471.60

Care staff mix is an uncertain variable determined by ward policy. However, variations in staff mix do not affect relative costs of care across the wards. In all cases the residents of Ward 3 and Ward 4 are the most expensive to care for and the residents of Ward 1 and Ward 2 are the cheapest.

The present mix [i] with a 70% occupancy level lies close to the mean of the care costs generated in the sensitivity analysis in Ward 2 and Ward 4, suggesting it to be a suitable representative measure of the cost of the provision of care staff when uncertainty surrounds both future staffing and occupancy levels. The mean cost of Ward 3 is lower than the cost of care staff calculated at mix [i] and a 70% occupancy level due to the higher occupancy level (83%) at the time of cost collection which generates smaller range, and therefore a lower mean.

Table 7.9
A summary of the sensitivity of costs to staff mix
and occupancy rates

Ward	Cost at 70% and mix [i] £	Size of range £	Matrix Mean £
1	320.46*		
2	359.21	126.40	360.30
3	432.76	108.07	388.17
4	453.76	159.30	440.30

*at current occupancy level

The final comparison is the number of staff on the ward compared to the number of residents. Assuming occupancy rates of 70% (except Ward 1), the ratios of staff to clients vary considerably across wards. In Ward 1, the staff to client ratio is 0.6, and in wards 2, 3 and 4 the staff to client ratios are 0.53, 0.87 and 0.95 respectively. As might be expected higher ratios are identified on the wards housing the residents with the highest psychiatric ratings (eg as rated in the Krawiecka Rating Scale) and, more pertinently for community care comparisons, the lowest dependency rating on the REHAB scale. The results of this sensitivity analysis support the findings of Wright (1987) and Marks (1985) that in order for a real investigation concerning the efficiency of the allocation of nurses to wards to be made, it is necessary to determine the optimum mix of staff for caring for that group of clients. In the absence of such information the cost figures at current staffing levels will be taken forward and used for comparative purposes.

Community care scheme costs

Much concern has been expressed that community care is a cheap alternative releasing the government from any responsibility of care provision for the mentally ill (Herman and Green, 1991). Hence the second phase of the evaluation program is to identify and measure, the costs of

180

resources used by the same clients following discharge to the different types of community care used in North Wales.

Over the course of the evaluation study community care placements have been found for 34 of the original cohort of 63 individuals. As described in chapter 3 they have been placed in a variety of settings: nine are in a ten person home (Community Care Scheme 1 - CCSI), fifteen are in five three person homes (Community Care Scheme 2 - CCSII), six are in social services and private care homes (Community Care Scheme 3 - CCS III), and four moved into family or independent living situations. Less information has been gained for those in independent living. The following analysis looks at the three care schemes, independent living information is given later.

The costs for CCS I are based on a 10 person home containing self-contained flats for 1,2 or 3 persons, a communal lounge for staff and residents, and staff areas, CCS I is managed by MIND and funded by a housing association.

The costs for CCS II are based on a housing scheme which comprises five self-contained houses, each giving a home to three individuals. Each house has 2 bedrooms (one shared) for the residents, and one bedroom for sleep-in-staff. The aim of the scheme is for residents to be able to lead a normal life in a 'normal' house. Twenty-four hour care staff cover is provided and staff share living facilities with residents.

The costs for CCS III are based on an example of a privately run nursing home for the mentally ill. CCS III has 22 residents; each resident has their own room and use of a communal kitchen, bathroom and lounge facilities.

Table 7.10
Outline of sample client characteristics

Characteristics			CCS I	CCS II	CCS III
Sample			9	15	6
Size of example home		9	5 x 3	22	
Age (years)	-	Mean	47.9	66.1	57.6
	-	S.D.	8.1	6.6	16.3
	-	Range	36-64	56-77	35-70
Sex	-	Male	7	14	12
	-	Female	2	1	
Length of present stay in hospital	-	Mean	10.9	27.4	21.8
	-	S.D.	11.5	12.9	17.2
	-	Range	0.4-30	8-47	3-45
Total number of years Hospitalised	-	Mean	16.4	32.7	25.7
	-	S.D.	13.4	8.3	18.0
	-	Range	3-35	19-46	4-45

181

The residents of these community schemes are of varying backgrounds. Table 7.10 shows the difference in client characteristics across the sample. The youngest clients are in CCS I, the oldest in CCS II, while residents of CCS III are spread in a range over the two. CCS I had the shortest mean present length of stay in hospital and the fewest years of hospitalisation, while CCS II has the longest mean present stay in hospital and most years of hospitalisation. CCS III has a larger standard deviation for total years hospitalised which indicates the more varied population.

The cost of care can vary with respect to clinical factors as well as demographic characteristics. The Krawiecka Rating Scale (KRS) psychiatric ratings and REHAB Total General Behaviour scores are used as indicators of psychiatric and social functioning, as reported by (Mitchell et al., this volume). The residents of CCS I, CCS II and CCS III exhibit different levels of symptom severity and varying dependency levels. The older, more institutionalised residents in CCS II exhibit very low rates of depression, anxiety, coherent delusions and hallucinations, while the relatively younger members of CCS I have more florid symptoms. The more active symptoms displayed by the younger individuals were reflected in higher costings in the hospital setting. The dependency level scores indicate that residents of CCS II and CCS III are less able to look after themselves than the residents of CCS I.

Collection of community costs

The resources used are classified in the same manner as those in the hospital: care staff services, external services, general services, personal consumption, and capital costs. Cost information was gained from interviews with the managers of the homes, with the aid of a questionnaire (Garrod & Vick, 1992). Information regarding those in independent living is gained from the quality of life questionnaire as described by Barry and Crosby in chapter 6. The cost of care staff services incorporates the cost of employing the managers and the care staff, including employers' contributions to national insurance and superannuation schemes. These are costed as at end of March, 1991. External services are those professional services not supplied by the employees of the home. These include GP input, consultant psychiatrist time, community psychiatric nurse (CPN) visits, and use of social services day centres. It is assumed that the use of these services do not vary considerably among the residents in each home, and are calculated as an average of each home type. General services include water rates, heating/lighting, insurance, staff expenses/training, cleaning materials, registration fees, audit and legal fees, depreciation, secretary, cleaner, phone bills, postage, sundries, office furniture, furniture and fittings, bedding and linen, staff uniforms, kitchen equipment and food. Personal consumption, unlike in the hospital, is funded purely by the DSS. Each resident receives £11.40 a week for expenditure on cigarettes, clothes and other goods that are not provided by the home.

Capital costs are calculated according to the monetary or opportunity cost incurred by the home. In CCS I and CCS III the equivalent annual costs (EAC) of capital is calculated as an annual opportunity cost, in CCS II the figure used is the amount charged by the housing association as rent for the property. EAC are calculated for CCS II for comparison purposes, but not used in the final costings.

Care staff services

The three homes have totally different staffing policies, made up of varying grades, numbers and payscales of care staff. CCS I has a staff to client ratio of 1.0. There is a key-worker responsible for each client. The staff comprises of a manager, a deputy manager, two senior project workers, six part-time project workers and an employment trainee. Each CCS II has a staff to client ratio of 1.6. Each house has the whole time equivalent (WTE) of 4.8 community support workers. CCS III has a staff to client ratio of 0.9. The staff are more qualified than those in CCS I and CCS II. There are 5 registered mental nurses (RMN), 2 state enrolled nurses (SEN), 15 care assistants and one manager (also a RMN) employed in CCS III. CCS III also employs 1.5 WTE cooks and 2.0 WTE domestics for communal cooking and cleaning. These variations in characteristics have produced large differences in the costs of maintaining clients in these homes, as highlighted in Table 7.11.

Table 7.11
Average costs for community care provision

	CCS I pw/resident £	CCS I pw/resident %	CCS II pw/resident £	CCS II pw/resident %	CCS III pw/resident £	CCS III pw/resident %
Care Staff Services	195.72	52.10	426.95	68.70	211.28	59.98
External Services	10.85	2.89	10.69	1.72	9.85	2.80
General Services	114.19	30.40	89.81	14.45	103.54	29.40
Personal Consumption	11.40	3.03	11.40	1.83	11.40	3.24
Rent/EAC of capital	43.47	11.57	82.65	13.30	16.15	4.59
Total Cost	375.63	100.00	621.50	100.00	352.23	100.00

The staff in the various homes are paid on different scales, either the National Joint Council (NJC) scale or the NHS scale. The care staff in CCS I are on the NJC, and CCS II and CCS III are on NHS. The impact of these differences shown in Table 7.12. Grade 11 staff (the lowest on NJC) are paid more than grade A staff (the lowest on NHS) whilst doing a similar job. The NJC scale 'grade 18' is included in Table 7.12 as care staff on the NJC scale are undergoing pay settlement discussions which may set the minimum wage at scale 18. The imminent new wage settlement will cause the cost per resident in CCS I to increase from £195.72 to at least £236.79.

The different salary and staffing policies of the three home types are set out in Table 7.13. The figures indicate that staffing levels have a greater impact (CCS II has a 77.8% higher staffing level than CCS III) on care staff service costs than do salary levels (CCS II has a 36.6% higher average salary cost per staff member than CCS I).

Table 7.12
Results of sensitivity analysis of influence of care staff grades

Community Care Scheme	Present Care Services Costs £	Replace with: NJC grades Grade 11 £	Grade 18 £	Grade 27 £	NHS grades Grade A £	Grade G £
I	195.72	194.22	236.79	305.89	143.83	318.93
II	398.67*	310.75	378.86	489.43	230.13	510.29
II	211.28	176.56	215.226	278.09	130.75	289.94

*These staff costs do not include non-care participant management

Table 7.13
Average cost of one member of staff in community care

Community Care Scheme	Staff-client Ratio	A.C. of staff /Resident	A.C. of one staff Member
I	1.00	195.72	195.72
II	11.60	398.67	249.17
III	0.90	199.04	221.16

However any effects are magnified because CCS II has both the highest staff-client ratio and average salary cost per staff member. Each scheme also has a different management structure (Table 7.14).

Table 7.14
Management costs

Community Care Scheme	W.T.E. No. of Mgmnt	Mgmnt Cost Per Week Per Individual	No. of Individuals per staff member	No. Managers Manager	Cost of one WTE
I	2.0	61.82	10	0.25	30.91
II	1.25	28.28	15	0.05	22.62
III	1.0	14.66	22	0.05	14.66

CCS I has 2 managers who are also care staff, CCS II has 1.25 WTE external staff who are also community psychiatric nurses (CPNs) for the unit, and CCS III has 1 manager who is also involved in provision of care. The management of CCS I and CCS III participate in active care in the home alongside their management duties. To eliminate any double counting it is assumed that the amount of time spent managing versus caring is 50% in both CCS I and CCS III. The actual cost of management is then approximately £30 in CCS I, £30 in CCS II, and £7 in CCS III. The average cost of management also shows how management are paid on different salary scales.

Capital costs

Due to the financing of the projects, capital costs vary quite considerably between the different care homes. CCS I is funded by a partnership between a housing association and voluntary organisation (MIND). The housing association provides the funding for the purchase and modernisation of the home, while the voluntary organisation provides the staff to manage the home. The housing association does not charge a rent for the property, just a nominal amount for upkeep and management services. This is subtracted from the special needs management allowance (SNMA) which the residents of the home are entitled to from the Welsh Office, via the housing association. CCS II was set up by the management of a housing association in collaboration with the health authority. The housing association funds the homes and their update, and charges the residents of the homes the equivalent of repayments for a 100% mortgage over 25 years. CCS III was purchased and updated privately: the owners provide the mortgage payments from the fees of the home. Total capital costs were available for all homes. The costs used in the analysis are equivalent annual costs for CCS I and CCS III, and rent charged for CCS II.

Table 7.15
Capital costs

Community Care Scheme	Cost/Resident p.w. £	% of Total Cost £
I [EAC]	43.47	11.57
II [RENT]	82.65	14.45
III [EAC]	6.15	4.59

From hospital care to community care

A comparison of the cost of care in hospital and community reveals an interesting change in the relative costs of caring for different types of clients. In hospital the older long stay residents (OLSR) from Ward 1 and Ward 2 cost less to care for than the newer long stay residents (NLSR) of Ward 3 and Ward 4. Levels of functioning vary between the residents of

185

the four wards and are seen as a significant contributory factor in the cost of care. Residents of Ward 1 and Ward 2 exhibit few active psychiatric symptoms, while residents of Ward 3 and Ward 4 show more florid symptoms requiring more psychiatric care input.

Age is highly correlated with psychiatric symptoms and hence may have an influence on the cost of care provision. Residents of Ward 1 and Ward 2 have mean ages of 68 and 61.2 years, and residents of Ward 3 and Ward 4, 44.8 and 39.5 years respectively. These age differences coincide with the variation in symptoms. Older psychiatric patients tend to exhibit less florid psychiatric symptoms and are physically less active - hence they require less intense rehabilitation. In fact, there appears to be little active rehabilitation work at all in either Ward 1 or Ward 2. The younger psychiatric patients, on the other hand, are more physically active and require more rehabilitation input.

The transfer from hospital into the various community care schemes causes large changes in cost and quality of care. The transfers are summarised in Figure 7.1. Those from the cheapest ward (Ward 1) moved into CCS II (the most expensive care type). The residents from Ward 2, Ward 3 and Ward 4 moved into CCS I and CCS III which were significantly cheaper than CCS II. The cost estimations have shown OLSP to cost more to care for in the community than the NLSP, whilst in hospital they had cost less. Both client characteristics and institutional factors may influence the costs of care. A comparison of costs for a particular set of individuals in hospital with the cost of care for the same set in the community settings should help identify the cost impact of care provision decisions rather than client needs.

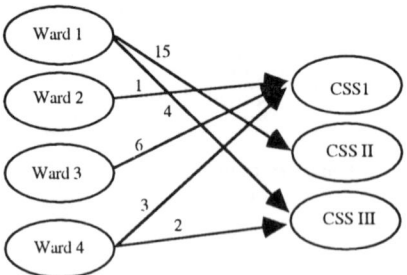

Figure 7.1: Movement of clients from hospital wards to community care homes

From ward 1 to community care scheme II

A comparison of Ward 1 and CCS II costs (Table 7.16) reveals that community care is roughly twice as expensive as hospital care. The majority of this difference occurs due to higher staffing and rental costs.

Table 7.16
Breakdown of total cost for ward 1 and community care scheme II

| | Ward I | | CCS II | |
	Cost per Week	% of Total Cost	Cost per Week	% of Total Cost
Care Staff Services	151.61	47.31	426.95	68.70
External Services	8.40	2.62	10.69	1.72
General Services	133.79	41.75	89.81	14.45
Personal Consumption	12.99	4.05	11.40	1.83
Rent	13.67	4.27	82.65	13.30
Total Cost	320.46	100.00	621.50	100.00

Care staff services

Care staff cost differences may be a result of staff grades, staff: client ratios or salary levels. When in hospital care (Ward 1) there were 15 staff caring for 26 individuals, giving a staff to client ratio of 0.6. In community care (CCS II) there is a staff to client ratio of 1.6, totalling 4.8 staff for the three individuals in each house. In ward 1 the staff mix is 1 G, 1 F, 6 E's and 5 B's; in CCS II, care staff are employed at grade C equivalents. Despite this difference in staff mix the average cost per member of staff is very similar: £252.68 for hospital staff and £249.17 for CCS II. Thus it is apparent that the staff to resident ratio is the main contributing factor to care staff services cost differences.

When the duties of the care staff in each care situation are analysed with respect to the REHAB TGB scores, an interesting relationship arises. In hospital Ward 1 the residents are provided with help for dressing, washing etc., with external services providing what little active rehabilitation there was. In CCS II the care staff provide active rehabilitation - encouraging participation with cooking, cleaning and other every day chores. A comparison of REHAB scores shows a large decrease in general behaviour scores from 72.14 (doubtful if patient could live outside) to 63.23 (could only live outside with much tolerance and supervision). This fall in REHAB TGB scores is likely to be due to the increase in input from the staff, and the opportunity to practice skills more frequently within the home (see chapter 3).

Between Ward 1 and CCS II, the main cause of variation in cost is the ratio of staff to residents. This could have one of two explanations. It may be that due to the larger size of Ward 1, economies of scale enable the provision of care with less staff, and therefore less cost. However, improvement in REHAB scores in the community setting would suggest that the higher cost in CCS II is due to increased, and more appropriate, care input.

External services

Any change in the use of external services can have important implications for local amenities in community settings. External service provision costs £8.40 per resident per week in Ward 1, and £10.69 in CCS II. The difference is not very large but there are differences in services provided. External services staff input includes medical staff such as the consultant psychiatrist, SHO/GP and psychologist visits. The residents have more input from external services staff once they are situated in the community than they had while they were in hospital. The residents of CCS II have regular checkups with the consultant and they visit the GP. The managers of the scheme are qualified community psychiatric nurses (CPN), thus CPN costs are implicit in management costs.

Occupational therapy input was available in the hospital, as part of its residents were able to work on the hospital farm previous to the running down of the hospital. Occupational therapy is provided by the care staff in CCS II as part of day-to-day care. Transfer of occupational therapy costs has occurred from external services to care staff services. This might explain the increase in staff input and costs. Residents are actively involved in household chores as part of their therapy. An art club, run by the social services, is attended by some members of the care scheme. The additional cost is borne out of weekly housekeeping costs.

The main amenities that will require extra facilities when clients are moved to the community will be the local GP practice and social service facilities.

General services

General services are the largest cost in the ward next to staffing. The cost of general services is £133.79 per resident per week, in CCS II it costs £89.81. The difference between the hospital and in the community is due to the overheads of running a large hospital. This explains approximately £34 of the difference. The main other difference lies in food and catering costs. In hospital specialist catering staff are employed to do the cooking; in CCS II the care staff do the cooking with the residents if possible, hence a lower cost. Again this is an example of a transfer cost. Catering costs are transferred from general services to care staff services. A similar explanation is available for the domestic/cleaning input as there are no domestic staff employed in CCS II.

Capital costs

Capital costs are largely determined by the funding organisation in charge of the home. CCS II residents are charged a rent of £86.65 per week by the housing association funding the purchase of the homes while the hospital capital costs are based on a 60 year life, with a 5% discount rate. An equivalent annual cost was also calculated over 25 years, the equivalent of a typical mortgage for both care situations. However, as Table 7.17 shows, when EAC are calculated over 60 and 25 years CCS II is still more expensive. This is due to economies of scale as a hospital for 300 people will not cost 100 times as much as a house for 3 people.

Table 7.17
Capital costs

	EAC@60 yrs. £	EAC@25 yrs. £	Rent £
Ward 1	13.67	18.38	N/A
CCS II	26.06	35.04	82.65

Also at the time the mortgage funding of the home was taken out interest rates and mortgage rates were high and the rent has therefore been set at a high level by the housing association. Unfortunately, the capital costs for CCS II have been caught in the high interest rates of the 1990s and as they have fallen the rent has not, due to government policy towards housing associations.

Summary

Ward 1 provides care more cheaply than CCS II. This is due to a lower input of resources, which, according to the KRS psychiatric ratings and REHAB TGB scores, results in psychiatric well-being of a lower standard. The community costs are higher due to more staff input, and capital costs. These are two variables which are predominantly governed by decisions which may be only indirectly influenced by client characteristics. Care staff input has to be relatively high in order to provide 24 hour care for three people in a home, and the capital costs are high due to the funding arrangements of the home.

From wards 2,3 and 4 to community care scheme I

Table 7.18
Cost of care in hospital and community care scheme I

Care Setting		Total Cost of Care
Hospital:	Ward 2	359.21
	Ward 3	432.77
	Ward4	543.64
	Weighted Ave.Mean	458.68
Community Care Scheme I		375.63

The residents of CCS 1 were previously living in wards 2,3 and 4 of the hospital. The difference in hospital and community care costs in this instance is not as wide as between Ward 1 and CCS II. CCS I is cheaper than Wards 3 and 4, and slightly more expensive, £10 per week per person, than Ward 2 (Table 7.18). If a weighted mean is taken (of the 10 residents in CSS 1 one came from Ward 2, six from Ward 3 and three from Ward 4) CCS I (£375.63) is cheaper than the hospital (£458.68).

As in the previous case, the breakdown of total costs (Table 7.19) shows care staff services as the major contributing factor to the differences in costs.

Table 7.19
Breakdown of costs from wards 2,3, 4 to community care scheme I

	Ward 2 £/w	Ward 3 £/w	Ward 4 £/w	Weighted Average	Community Care Scheme 1 £/w
Care Staff Services	181.50	245.05	337.06	266.30	195.72
External Services	9.37	24.21	32.90	25.33	10.85
General Services	142.41	137.62	151.44	142.25	114.19
Personal Consumption	19.44	19.40	15.75	18.31	11.40
Rent	6.49	6.49	6.49	6.49	43.47
Total Cost	359.21	432.77	543.64	458.68	375.63

Care staff services

The hospital wards had a very similar make up of qualified and lesser qualified staff to that of CCS 1. Each ward had 3-5 staff above grade D, and the remainder are less qualified, while the home has 4 qualified staff and 6 unqualified. As qualifications are fairly similar, the difference in costings must be explained by a difference in staff pay scales. The employees of the home are paid on the social services National Joint Council (NJC) scale. The staff of the hospital are paid for night duty, while staff in CCS I are not. This makes a large difference in salary costs. Clearly care staff cost difference caused by pay scale differences are institution and not needs driven.

External services

The use of external services has fallen for wards 3 and 4 from £24.21 and £32.90 respectively to £10.85 per resident per week in CCS I. The cost for ward 2 has risen from £9.37 to £10.85 since leaving the hospital.

There is a large variation in costs between each setting. A number of factors can explain this variation. In hospital the clients had occasional consultant visits, Senior House Officer (SHO) visits attending any physical illness, and occupational therapy (the major contributor to cost). Once they moved into the community the services utilised changed and residents used services such as GP, social services day centres, and have more frequent contact with their consultant.

The residents no longer received specific occupational therapy as it is provided on a more informal day-to-day basis by the care staff. This is a transfer of costs from external services to care staff services. Therefore, although staff costs rise the cost of occupational therapy disappears as the staff are employed to rehabilitate the residents. In order to directly compare, it would be necessary to isolate occupational therapy from the rest of care provided by care staff. However, it would appear that occupational therapy input has fallen in the community setting, particularly for Ward 3 and 4 residents.

Summary

The comparison of the cost of care and resources used in Ward 2, Ward 3 and Ward 4 versus CCS I has shown some interesting relationships. CCS I on average is cheaper than the hospital wards. The main reasons for this appear to be the lower pay scales for community workers and lower costs of general services. Neither of these items, of course, are needs driven and highlight the importance of centralised strategic decision making on cost structures.

From ward 1 and 4 to community care scheme III

Table 7.20
Breakdown of costs from ward 1 to community care scheme III

	Ward 1		Community Care Scheme III	
	£/w	% of TC	£/w	% of TC
Care Staff Services	151.61	47.31	211.28	59.98
External Services	8.40	2.61	9.85	2.80
General Services	133.79	39.65	103.54	29.40
Personal Consumption	12.99	4.05	11.40	3.24
Rent	13.67	4.27	16.15	4.59
Total Cost	320.46	100.00	352.23	100.00

The third comparison is between the hospital wards and a private care home. Four residents moved from Ward 1 and 2 from Ward 4, but the private care home under analysis houses one resident from Ward 1.

The difference in costs of care between a resident in Ward 1 and CCS III, is not very large (Table 7.20) but the constituent parts are quite different.

Care staff services

Community Care Scheme III has a staff to client ratio of 0.9, and ward 1 has a ratio of 0.6. If both care settings are staffed with a ratio of 1.0 staff per client the cost of care becomes £421.53 for ward 1, and £375.71 for Community Care Scheme III. As staff in both care settings are paid on NHS scales it appears that Ward 1 was staffed by higher grade personnel.

External services

Provision of external services for residents of ward 1 costs £8.40 per resident per week, and in CCS III it costs £9.85. Although cost does not change, the resident makes more use of services such as the local GP and consultant psychiatrist when situated in the community. The duties of a community psychiatric nurse are provided by the staff in the home (another transfer cost from external services to care staff services). Residents of CC III have entertainment provided in the home which is included in the duties of the care staff's work.

Summary

The provision of care staff services varies between the two homes. CCS III employs 0.9 staff per resident while Ward 1 employs 0.6 staff per client. This explains some of the difference in costs. The rest of the difference is explained by the higher grading of staff in Ward 1. External services costs are similar and appear to vary more in the amount of input rather than the cost of the input. General services are generally cheaper in the home.

From hospital to independent living

Of the 63 individuals in the initial cohort of movers, 4 moved into independent living situations. The costs of care for these people are not included in the main costings analysis as they are not very comprehensive. Costs were collected for DSS money, GP, Psychiatrist and CPN visits and rent.

Table 7.21
Total cost of care for independent living

Individual	£/week
A	85.43
B	89.60
C	51.06
D	101.01

The costs incurred for these people are much lower than those actually in care homes as they do not require care staff input (Table 7. 21).

Individuals A and C have no rent to pay as they live with relatives. Individual B has no contact with a consultant. Individual B and D are awarded rent allowance payable to the council for the council flats. Social work is infrequent and information is hard to gain on this.

Although these costs are not very detailed, they are interesting for comparisons of costs for individuals who are no longer in an official care setting. They highlight just how much of total costs of residential care is governed by care staff services.

Explanatory variables of cost

Knapp, Beecham, Anderson, Dayson, Leff, Margolium, O'Driscoll and Wills (1990) explore variations in community costs in comparison to baseline hospital characteristics of hospital leavers. Using cost per week as the dependent variable, and the full range of patient data as explanatory factors, ordinary least squares multiple regression is used to investigate any association. The regression provided an equation explaining 38% of the observed cost variation. The main predictors are found to be age at time of hospital assessment, current length of hospital stay, total time ever in psychiatric hospital, proportion of life spent in hospital and social functioning as measured by the Social Behaviour Schedule. They use this equation to show that assessments of patient characteristics in hospital give adequate information regarding client needs and that the equation can be used to predict more than a third of the variations in community costs.

A similar exploration was undertaken with the costs from this study. As in Knapp et al. (1990), cost per resident per week is used as the dependent variable whilst the explanatory variables are age in years, 'general life satisfaction' as measured on the Quality of Life Schedule, and 'attitudes to discharge', (as described in chapter 6), length of present hospital stay, REHAB TGB scores and scores for KRS. Ordinary least squares multiple regression produces one significant variable, with a p-value of less than 0.05 namely, 'age in years'. Age is found to be able to predict 27.3% of the total cost of care in the community.

A second regression is run with different explanatory variables. The second regression is an adapted version of the first, in order to attempt to replicate the work by Knapp et al. (1990) more closely. The variables in the first regression are multiplied by 'age in years' and 'total years in hospital'. However, again the only significant variable is 'age in years'. A full summary of the results is provided in Garrod and Vick (1992).

The results produced by the regression are not unexpected for two principle reasons. Throughout the analysis it has been evident that the older residents of the sample have moved into the more expensive care homes. Secondly, the cost data collected was on a ward or institutional level and not client specific. This was partly due to a lack of individual client costings, which are so difficult to achieve, but can be defended by the extensive discussions with community care managers who believed that care inputs were utilised on a home rather than client basis.

With only three observations of the dependent variable, regression analysis would not seem to be an appropriate form of analysis. The regressions were only run for comparative purposes with the results of Knapp et al. Their study revealed few significant associations between costs and accommodation type. They did, however find that residential care and staffed group homes are more expensive than other care forms and that independent living is the cheapest form of care.

In the TAPS study the number of home types was greater than 30, while our study there were only three. It is likely that the TAPS data has sufficient variation in community care scheme that this is not a dominant factor. In our more restricted sample, institutional factors might be playing a more important role in driving community care costs. The TAPS study costed care provision for clients once they moved into existing care provision facilities. In the majority of cases in the NWH study community care facilities had to be created in order to care for the clients. As these facilities were both small and new there is a sense in which individual client costings are unrealistic. The general philosophy behind the community care provided is to integrate the clients into social activity and behaviour such that group activity is encouraged. This leads to average costings being the most appropriate figures to use for comparative purposes. This means, of course, that institutional or planning factors are likely to play a dominant role in costing community care.

Also the explanatory variables identified by Knapp et al., are precisely the factors which show high correlation in our sample. For example, the older clients who, on average, had greater measures of current length of stay, total time ever in psychiatric hospital, proportion of life spent in hospital and poorer levels of social functioning were housed in CCS II, the most expensive care form. Thus, although individual patient characteristics may not be identified as explanatory variables in our study they are implicit in the decision taken about the type of care form required and the homes to which clients are sent. What the comparison of the results from the two studies does highlight is the difficulty in isolating client needs driven costs from those which result from institutional decisions regarding appropriate care forms, staffing levels and financing methods.

Funding

The source of funding for mental health care. The provision of mental health care for deinstitutionalised clients involves various agencies providing services. The costing exercise has disguised some interesting differences in the agencies providing a service in different care settings. If health authority costs alone are collected the movement of patients to the community would result in a fall in the cost of care. In hospital the main providers are the NHS, with a 'pocket money' contribution from the DSS. Once in the community the providers are more diverse, and vary between the type of care schemes. In CCS I the principle contributor is the DSS, who provide the allowance to cover 48% of costs of care, other contributors include, the housing association, local health authority, and the NHS. In CCS II the principle contributor is the local health authority, with other contributions from social services, the DSS and the NHS. CCS III is funded predominantly by the DSS, with minimal contribution from the owner. These sources of funds are summarised in Table 7.22.

It is evident from Table 7.22, that there are many agencies providing care for individuals when they move into the community. There is a transfer of costs from the NHS to local health authorities, the Department of Social Security, the Department of Environment, and other agencies. It is possible that some of the costings are affected by the resource provider. As a first attempt to investigate this question, organisational inputs in each care setting are examined more closely.

North Wales Hospital, wards 1-4

Table 7.22
Source of funds for care

Types of Residential Provision	NHS Hospital	CSS I	CSS II	CSS III	Independent Living
1. National Health Service					
Health and Community Service	X	X	X	-	-
Family Practitioner Comm.	-	-	X	-	X
2. Local Auth. Soc. Services Dept.					
Day Care	-	-	X	-	X
3. Dept. of Social Security					
Income Support	X	X	X	X	X
Housing Benefit	-	-	-	-	X
Board and Lodgings	-	X	X	X	X
Attendance Allowance	-	X	X	X	X
4. Dept. of Environment					
Housing Association Grants	-	X	X	-	-
SNMA	-	-	-	-	X

As discussed previously, the four wards are situated in a NHS hospital and are funded by the government. The services provided in the hospital, eg occupational therapy, are run by the NHS and as such are funded by them. There are small inputs from social workers, when resettlement discussions are undertaken - but this is not within the ordinary care routine. Hence, costs are one hundred per cent NHS funded.

The weekly costs borne by the various agencies for the community care schemes are set out in table 7.23.

Table 7.23
Source and value of funding for the community care schemes

Source of Funds	CCS I		CCS II		CCSS III		Independent Living	
	£/Week	%	£/Week	%	£/Week	%	£/Week	£
DSS	181	48.3	181	29.2	286	81	78	77
Housing Association: SNMA	44	11.7						
Capital	39	10.4						
Local Health Authority	102	27.2						
NHS	9	2.4	11	1.8	10	4	26	23
Social Services			2	0.3				
Local Authority			426	68.7				
Owners					56	15		
Total	375	100	620	100	352	100	104	100

Discussion and conclusion

The aim of this study is to identify the resources used by various forms of community and hospital based care for long-term psychiatric clients in North Wales; to measure the costs of those resources; to compare the costs of hospital based with community based care; to determine costs falling to different agencies; and to identify factors which may influence the cost of care in community settings.

Work by Knapp and Beecham (1990a) points to a cost of care which can be forecast from client characteristics and, by implication, client needs and finds no association between the type of institution and the total cost of care. In the NWH study a similar multiple regression analysis shows only one significant predictor of costs: age in years. This is not surprising as the older residents are placed in the most expensive home and younger residents in the cheaper home. This suggests that perhaps it is not the needs of the clients directly that determine the cost, but rather the placement of the client to the 'appropriate' care home type.

Unlike the TAPS example, where clients were moved to existing facilities, the community care provision provided in North Wales in CCS I and CCS II were new and specially designed for the population of clients moving to the community. Thus whilst client characteristics and needs will have been taken into account in the design of these facilities it will be institutional decisions regarding the care form type which will dominate in any cost analysis. A statistical tautology exists in the case where average costs of care facilities are regressed against individual client characteristics and care home type but in the North Wales experience it reflects both the philosophy and practice in the new facilities.

It is clear that a significant determinant of the cost of community care is the decision by authorities to provide certain types of homes, including the size of the home, the care staff employed and the funding raised for the provision of the home. Results of assessments of psychiatric well-being and quality of life (see chapters 4 and 6 of this volume) view that appropriate planning decisions were taken. However, few conclusions can be drawn about the economic efficiency of the provision of such care due to the limited range of facilities available to accommodate clients of similar needs.

The method of client placement can be determined in three ways; by client needs, by client characteristics, or by policy decisions of health authorities. A needs driven policy would enable a predictive equation to be derived to forecast future costs based on the needs of the clients. Similarly, a characteristics driven policy would enable the production of a predictive equation to match clients to a care form and hence predict costs. Such a predictive equation is provided by Knapp and Beecham (1990). However, in the case of a policy driven system, a predictive equation is difficult to identify as client characteristics might only indirectly provide an indication of the costs of the care provided.

The results of the NWH study lead us to believe that the cost of care for the mentally ill in North Wales is predominantly policy driven. The cost analysis produces staff make-up and size of home as the main determinants of cost, which are policy driven decisions. It is a very large assumption that provision matches need, especially as only rudimentary needs assessment has been undertaken. When regressing the cost of care with respect to client characteristics, it is implicit that the clients have been placed in the most appropriate care form.

It appears that little work has been done to investigate, and cost, the needs of clients as opposed to costing facilities or services already supplied. As stated by Matthews (1971);

A need for medical care exists when an individual has an illness or disability for which there is effective and acceptable treatment or care. It can be defined either in terms of the type of illness or disability causing the need, or of the treatment, or facilities, for treatment required to meet it. A demand for care exists when an individual considers that he has a need and wishes to receive care. Utilisation occurs when an individual actually receives care. Need is not necessarily expressed as demand, and demand is not necessarily followed by utilisation, while, on the other hand, there can be demand and utilisation without real underlying need for the particular service used.

The method of allocation of clients to care forms is, therefore, crucial. Hafner and an der Heiden (1989) state, 'Estimates of the cost of care are realistic only if patients' needs are being adequately met'. Need is defined on the basis of problems in individual functioning, rather than diagnostic levels; a need is present where a patient's functioning falls below, or threatens to fall below, some minimum specified level and this is due to some remediable cause. Buckingham and Ludbrook (1989) look at 'intra-client' variations in cost and show that needs may change over time as should care provision. This is likely to be a characteristic of the NWH study, particularly in CCS I and CCS II. Improvements in social and domestic skills are only finite and the need for current staffing and occupational therapy policies may be short lived. This, of course, would have significant implications on long-term community care costs. The authors therefore caution the direct use of cost figures identified in this study. Rather they would highlight the collection processes used and the institutional pressures which drive the absolute cost figures. At a more general level it is clear from this study that care can be as cheap or expensive as policy makers wish. A change from large institution to community based care facilitie will not, of itself, influence the cost of care provision. What it does do is offers policy makers the ability to reconsider the nature and quality of care provided and thus improve the quality of life of long stay psychiatric clients.

References

Bohm, P. (1987), *Social Efficiency: A Concise Introduction to Welfare Economics*. Macmillan Education

Buckingham, K. and Ludbrook, A. (1989), *Costing Community Care; Some Problems and Proposals*. HERU University of Aberdeen. Discussion Paper 06/89

Conroy, J. and Bradley (1985), *Penhurst Longitudinal Study, A Report of 5 Years Research and Analysis*. Philadelphia, PA: Temple University.

Davies, L. (1987), *Quality Costs and an Ordinary Life*. London: Kings Fund Project Paper, no 67.

Department of Health and Social Security (1985), *Social Services Committee Report on Community Care*. London: HMSO

Department of Health and Social Security (1983), *Care in Community*, London: HMSO

Garrod, N. and S Vick (1992), *Costing Care for the Mentally Ill: Causes and Outcomes* University of Wales, Bangor: Working Paper no. 92.6

Glennester, H. (1990), 'The Costs of Hospital Closure: Reproviding Services for the Residents of Darenth Park Hospital', *Psychiatric Bulletin,* Vol. 14, pp. 140-143.

Hafner, H. and Heiden, W. (1989a), 'The Evaluation of Mental Health Care Systems', *British Journal of Psychiatry,* Vol. 155, pp. 12-17.

Henderson, J. and Mooney, G. (1984), *Economic Principles of Applied Option Appraisal*. HERU University of Aberdeen. SOAP 1

Herman, D. and Green, J. (1991), *Madness:A Study Guide*. BBC Education Publication.

Hyde, C, Bridges, K., Goldberg, D., Lowson, K., Sterling, C, and Farragher, B. (1987), 'The Evaluation of a Hostel Ward, A Controlled Study using Modified Cost Benefit Analysis', *British Journal of Psychiatry* Vol. 151, pp. 805-812.

Klarman, H.E. (1974), 'Application of Cost-Benefit Analysis to the Health Services and the Special Case of Technological Innovation', *International Journal of Health Services,* Vol.4, No. 2

Korman, N. and Glennester, H. (1990), *Hospital Closure.* OUP.

Knapp, M. and Beecham, J. (1990a), 'Costing Mental Health Services', *Psychological Medicine*, Vol. 20, pp. 893-908.

Knapp, M. and Beecham, J. (1990b), 'The Cost-effectiveness of Community Care for former long-stay psychiatric hospital patients', in Scheffler and Rossiter, *Advances in Health Economics and Health Services Research* JAI Press 1990. Vol. 11, pp. 201-227.

Knapp, M., Beecham, J., Anderson, J. Dayson, D., Leff, J. Margolius, O. O'Driscoll, C. and Wills, W. (1990), 'The TAPS project 3: Predicting the Community Costs of Closing Psychiatric Hospitals', *The British Journal of Psychiatry,* Vol. 157, 661-670.

Mangen, S.P., Paykel, E.S., Griffith, Burchell and Mancini (1983), 'Cost Effectiveness of Community Psychiatric Nurses in outpatient care of neurotic patients', *Psychological Medicine ,* Vol. 13, pp. 407-416

Marks, I. (1985), 'Controlled Trials of Psychiatric Nurse Therapists in Primary Care', *British Medical Journal,* Vol. 290, pp.1181-1184.

Matthews, G.K. (1971), *Measuring Need and Evaluating Services.* Portfolio for Health, (ed.) G. McLachlan.

May, P.R.A. (1971), 'Cost Efficiency of Treatments for Schizophrenic Patients', *American Journal of Psychiatry,* 127:10.

Samuelson, P.A. (1976), Economies Tokyo: McGraw-Hill

Tansella, M. (1991), Community Based Psychiatry: Long-Term patterns of Care in South Verona (ed.),. *Psychological Medicine Monograph Supplement 19.* Cambridge University Press.

Weisbank, B.A. and Helming, M. (1980), 'What benefit analysis can and cannot do: The case of treating the mental ill', *Evaluation Studies Review Annual,* 604-621

Weisbrod, B.A., Test, M.A. and Stein, L.I. (1980), 'Alternative to Mental Hospital Treatment II Economic Benefit-Cost Analysis', *Archives of General Psychiatry.,* 37. April 1980

Williams, A. (1974), 'The Cost Benefit Approach', *British Medical Bulletin*, Vol. 30, No. 3

Wright, K.G. (1987), *Cost Effectiveness in Community Care.* CHC University of York. Discussion Paper 7.

Wright, K.G., Cairns, J.A., Snell, M.C. (1981), *Costing Care.* University of Sheffield Social Services Monograph, Research in Practice, Sheffield

Wright, K. and Haycox, A. (1985), *Costs of Alternative forms of NHS Care for Mentally Handicapped Persons.* CHE University of York. Discussion Paper 7.

Wykes, T. (1982), 'Hostel Ward for 'New' Long Stay', ...*Psychological Medicine Monograph Supplement,* 2, p. 55-97.

8 The development of community mental health services in North Wales: A research programme

Charles Crosby and Margaret M. Barry

Summary

The resettlement of patients from the North Wales Hospital forms part of a wider process of reorganising Mental Health Services in North Wales to provide local services delivered by community mental health teams. The establishment of such teams in Clwyd and Gwynedd is now well advanced. A research methodology which is being implemented by the Health Services Research Unit to evaluate the provision of community mental health services is outlined. This suggests the importance of placing assessment of individual need at the centre of community care. The assessment of client functioning is linked to the assessment of care practices and economic data collection in a research programme which will provide systematic, detailed information and care management and the cost-effectiveness of care packages for disadvantaged and vulnerable client groups. An outline of the proposed research programme is given in this chapter.

Introduction

The resettlement of long-stay patients from North Wales Hospital forms part of a larger reorganisation of mental health services in Clwyd and Gwynedd. Since 1948 the North Wales Hospital had been the focal point of mental health services for the counties of Clwyd and Gwynedd. The introduction of the Clwyd County Plan for Mental Illness Services (1991) and Mental Illness Services: A Strategy for Gwynedd (1992) was in response to objectives developed by the Welsh Office, which targeted the transfer of all mental health services away from hospital based provision to a community based pattern of care which would be focused on Community Mental Health Teams (CMHTs). The establishment of multi-disciplinary

201

CMHTs as the vehicle for delivery of services in the community had been anticipated in Gwynedd, notably by the early formation of the Arfon CMHT. The core members of the CMHTs currently developing in Clwyd and Gwynedd are workers in psychiatry, psychology, nursing, social work and occupational therapy. Other workers may include physiotherapists, dieticians, arts therapists and welfare rights advisors. In developing CMHTs in Clwyd collaboration was established between Clwyd Health Authority, Clwyd Social Services Department, Clwyd Mental Health Alliance and Clwyd Family Health Services Authority. The pathways for referral and the anticipated pattern of service provision are shown in Figure 8.1 (taken from Clwyd County Plan for Mental Illness Services, 1991).

In terms of referral, the General Practitioner clearly has a central role and this has led to the establishment of liaison by CMHTs with the primary care teams in the areas which they cover.

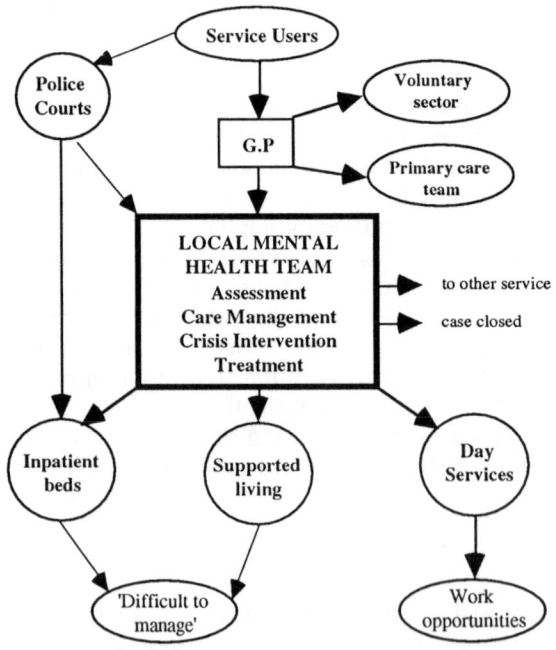

Figure 8.1
Adult illness: Pathways for referral

The establishment of a research response to these developments in service delivery was discussed at an early stage between the University College of North Wales, the Welsh Office and the relevant Health Authorities and Social Services Departments. A Research Advisory Group was established to assist in the development of an evaluation programme to complement the service changes. Such a research programme was seen as a natural development of the existing evaluation of resettlement from the North Wales Hospital (Crosby, et al., 1993).

The need for such evaluation research is strongly justified by the literature (Holloway et al., 1991; Huxley et al., 1990; Shepherd, 1990). The implementation of effective care management systems has yet to be more fully informed by research documenting its application to standard service provision and providing empirical evidence of its impact on users. Identifying the service needs of clearly defined client groups is a priority in order that service development and care planning may be successfully targeted. In particular, the needs of clients with long-term problems are prioritised, as studies (Sayce et al., 1991 and Goldie et al., 1989) show that community services frequently fail to meet the needs of vulnerable and disadvantaged people with long term severe disabilities. Patmore and Weaver (1991) address this problem and conclude that comprehensive mental health services have yet to be achieved and call for more detailed research on the needs of users, particularly the needs of the long term established clientele. Current policy identifies care management as a key coordinating mechanism for the delivery of community care to long-term clients who may require a range of dispersed services. However, as Huxley et al. (op. cit.) point out, the role of the care manager may be implemented differently and may have different meanings in different settings. Empirical evidence is needed regarding the effectiveness of different care management approaches and the extent to which they succeed in tailoring packages of care to individual needs and in producing positive outcomes for service users. Exploring the functioning of multidisciplinary teamwork and inter-agency collaboration in community mental health teams may also inform how care management evolves as the new services develop (Ryan et al., 1991). The costs of the provision of different care management packages to specific client groups also requires careful analysis. Previous research into the costs of supplying different forms of care for users of mental health services has encountered the problems of joint costs, (for example, Knapp and Beecham, 1990, and Korman and Glennerster, 1990). Other studies have had more success in identifying client characteristics with care management costs (Knapp et al., 1990) but all have highlighted the difficulties of dealing with joint and structural costs in their analyses. Using the projected client groups for the proposed research it will be possible to collect individual needs assessment and service utilisation data for each client and convert this into an individual cost. By costing needs rather than allocating institutional joint costs it will be possible to identify bilateral relationships between specific client characteristics and levels and types of costs. This type of information will prove a valuable input both for planning and budgetary purposes and serve as an objective assessment of care-form effectiveness.

203

The research samples will be drawn from the clients of four CMHTs (N=160) and from clients to be resettled from hospital (N = 63), giving a total of 223 cases. The research protocol will provide for a comprehensive package of assessments to be undertaken with members of the research cohorts, their principal formal carers and the service agency involved in providing care. The sample will be carefully structured to include representative proportions of different client groups, including:

1. acute cases referred to CMHTs
2. young chronic clients resident in the community
3. difficult to mange patients being resettled from hospital
4. old long-stay patients being resettled from hospital.

The development of a comparative research methodology will build upon the existing research protocol of the HSRU team (Crosby, Barry, Mitchell, Grant, Horrocks and Littlejohns, 1989) which has been successfully implemented with a cohort of patients being resettled from the North Wales Hospital. This methodology involves a repeated measures design in which data collected at baseline and a six months repeat assessment is used to provide controlled feedback of data to key workers and care managers. Assessment will then take place at eighteen months, again followed by controlled feedback, and 30 months, to assess the responsiveness of care management to needs assessment data collected by the research. This inter-active design makes the research unique.

The research will adopt a comparative approach to the four CMHTs, which represent different stages of development and patterns of service delivery. The effectiveness of CMHTs will be assessed against policy statements which state desired methods of operation and outcomes of management and care process. The All Wales Mental Illness Strategy (May, 1989) sets out a strategy framework to guide the development of a new pattern of mental health services. The following criteria are noted:

i) The main point of access to the specialist services for adult general psychiatry should be an identified member of the mental health team.
ii) Mental health teams should work closely and effectively with primary care teams.
iii) The mental health team should have a multi-disciplinary core of people most directly involved with the patient's programme of treatment, including medical, nursing, social work, psychology, occupational therapy and other professional groups supplementary to medicine.
iv) Staff should be appropriately trained and there should be sufficient manpower resources to allow the development of special expertise to which other team members could refer, and to provide out of hours cover.

v) Service delivery should be based on local circumstances and the extent to which need has been identified.

The research will examine the extent and character of internal team working, inter service relationships and collaboration. It will examine the extent to which the CMHTs carry a caseload of people who have serious mental health problems and evaluate the quality and quantity of the service which they receive. The pattern of referral and the characteristics of caseloads will be compared between CMHTs. A selection will be made from two client groups - young chronic clients (below the age of 40) and new referrals experiencing acute problems. The research will assess the psychiatric, social and behavioural and quality of life outcomes for clients matched for sex, age, diagnosis, length of contact with CMHT and total length of any periods of hospitalisation. It will relate outcomes to variations in care process and inputs between CMHTs. This comparative methodology will enable us to identify good practices which produce positive outcomes for the two client groups.

Selection of the research cohorts

1. Young adult chronic clients. Where no complete case register exists key workers' client caseloads will be collated.

Clients will be selected according to criteria of sex, age, diagnosis, length of contact with the community mental health team and total length of any periods of hospitalisation. Twenty clients in each of four CMHTs is the target number. If cases exceed this a random selection will take place from the pool of cases. Clients will be invited to participate in the research. A reserve list will be held where possible, in case of refusals.

2. Acute clients currently residing in the community.

Referrals to each team will be monitored for a six month period. Clients referred with an acute episode will be selected according to criteria of sex, age, diagnosis and total length of any periods of hospitalisation. Where possible a reserve list will be held in case of refusals. Twenty clients in each of four CMHTs is the target number.

The objective of these selection procedures is to obtain research cohorts which are matched between the four CMHTs.

Continuation of existing research

3 & 4. New long-stay patients and old long-stay patients.

Clients in this category have been resettled or are currently resident in North Wales hospital and will be resettled to the care of CMHTs by 1995, when the hospital will close. Three baseline assessments have already been undertaken with each patient remaining in hospital. They are the remainder of a continuing HSRU study (Crosby et al., 1993). The completion of this study will complement the work with CMHTs and will enable us to assess the success of the move from hospital to community care and to determine whether community care improves quality of life in comparison with hospital care.

Table 8.1
Main components of data collection for the community samples

Assessment of client functioning	Assessment of care practices	Economic data collection
psychiatric state *	documenting working models of care management *	checklist on type and nature of daily service inputs *
social and behabioural functioning *	assessing user involvement strategies *	apportioning costs to service elements *
quality of life *	needs case conference *	relating costs information to client characterstics
living conditions *	staff attitudes *	
needs assessment *	staff appraisal	
user evalution of service quality		

Data analysis will require a sophisticated approach. Multi-variate analysis will be used to carry out longitudinal repeated measures analysis of changes in client functioning and quality of life, care practices and related costs. The design of the study, with a comprehensive range of data being collected at repeated intervals, provides a unique opportunity to carry out a detailed investigation of the pattern of relationships between the care management process, client outcomes and cost measures.

Benefits of results

• The research will provide systematic, detailed information on effective care management and the cost effectiveness of care packages for important, disadvantaged and vulnerable client groups. It will inform and contribute significantly to good practice in care management for these groups and it will give guidance to policy makers on the most cost effective ways of securing health gains for clients with severe mental health problems.

- The repeat assessments in the community will provide information on the changing patterns of individual needs and will also permit an assessment of the responsiveness of the services to the identified needs of clients.
- The provision of firmly founded service costs will be of considerable value to service providers, purchasers, and policy makers in considering different management and service options and their associated resource effectiveness.
- Feedback of results from the research will enable the service providers to review progress, changing needs, and the resulting resource requirements and will inform the design of targeted services.
- The development of a standardised assessment package by the research team will make a significant contribution to practitioner assessment tools and will enable staff to become self-sufficient in respect of undertaking internal monitoring and evaluation.
- The dissemination of the findings from the evaluation of service developments in North Wales will provide valuable lessons that will inform mental health policy at a national as well as local level.

References

Crosby, C., Barry, M.M., Carter, M.F. and Lowe, C.F. (1993), 'Psychiatric rehabiliation and community care: resettlement from a North Wales Hospital,' *Health and Social Care* Vol. 1, 355-563.

Goldie, N., Pilgrim, D., Rogers, A. (1989), *Community Mental Health Centres: Policy and Practice.* London: Good Practices in Mental Health.

Holloway, F., McLean, E.K. and Robertson, J.A. (1991), 'Case management', *British Journal of Psychiatry,* 159, 142-148.

Huxley, P., Hagan, T., Hennelly, R. and Hunt, J. (1990), *Effective Community Mental Health Services,* Aldershot: Avebury.

Knapp, M. and Beecham, J. (1990), 'The cost effectiveness of community care for former long stay psychiatric hospital patients', *Advances in Health Economics and Health Services Research, 11,* 201-227.

Knapp, M., Beecham, J., Anderson, J., Dayson, D., Leff, J., Margolius, O., O'Driscoll, C. and Wills, W. (1990), 'The TAPS project 3: Predicting the community costs of closing psychiatric hospitals', *British Journal of Psychiatry, 157,* 661-670.

Korman, N. and Glennerster, H. (1990), *Hospital Closure.* Oxford University Press.

Patmore, C. and Weaver, T. (1991), *Community Mental Health Teams: Leassons for Planners and Managers.* Good Practices in Mental Health: London.

Ryan, P., Ford, R. and Clifford, P. (1991), 'Case management and community care', *Research and Development for Psychiatry.*

Sayce, L., Craig, T.K.J. and Boardman, A.P. (1991), 'The development of community mental health centres in the UK', *Social Psychiatry and Psychiatric Epidemiology, 26,* 14-20.

Shepherd, G. (1990), 'Case management', *Health Trends, 2,* 59-61.

9 Involving users in mental health services in the era of the word-processor and the database

David Healy

Summary

While the de-institutionalisation of psychiatric services continues at pace, many of the working models being transferred into the community derive from institutional settings and perpetuate an institutionalisation without walls. The Aberconwy Community Mental Health Team have worked on three strategies in order to combat this. These include, copying all clinic letters to general practitioners and others to patients. This involves a different style of letter writing rather than merely a photocopying exercise. The consequences of this are outlined. A second initiative has been to construct handouts on the various classes of medication and their side effects, which have been agreed by all team members. The rationale behind constructing such handouts and the impact of these handouts on patient care is outlined. Thirdly, an attempt has been made to record case information in a manner that makes more salient the need to collect information on the patients'/clients' own efforts to explain what has brought them to treatment, what apprehensions they have regarding treatment and what the consequences of prior treatment have been.

Introduction

Until quite recently psychological medicine has been dominated by the delivery of services within institutional settings. In these settings, technical expertise was largely vested in the institutions' medical officers. Nursing staff effectively filled custodial roles and there were few other staff, ancillary or paramedical. The keeping of clinical records was effectively the exclusive preserve of the medical profession.

The evolution of multidisciplinary working within institutional settings did little to change this. While other disciplines also began to take notes, a partition grew up between the various disciplines, which was graphically symbolised by the partitions within patient files separating medical from nursing, psychological, social work and occupational or other therapy notes, with little or no cross-talk between these bodies of information. Locked within filing-cabinets inaccessible to the patient, this information, in great part supplied by the patient, testified only to the power of the institutions over the individual.

With the development of community mental health teams, this mode of working has often simply transferred into the community. The different professions within the mental health teams keep entirely separate files. In general the medical file is still seen as being the only one of "substance", or at least of medico-legal import.

The practices of community mental health teams are sometimes castigated in terms of their fostering an institutionalisation without walls. The practice of record keeping, which has transferred straight from the older institutions into community settings without much modification, is one instance in which such covert institutionalisation may still be operative.

This is particularly the case as traditional practices are increasingly inappropriate in community mental health settings and teams, where there is a wide range of professional input and where increasingly most members of the team have higher qualifications. With the move into communities, therefore, it seems appropriate that new methods of record keeping be sought.

Furthermore, in psychiatry, more perhaps than in any other branch of medicine, a patient's record can subserve functions other than simply the medico-legal one. One of the goals of psychiatric treatment is to enlist the patient as a co-therapist. While this perhaps should also happen in other branches of medicine (Kleinman, 1988; Bursztajn et al., 1990), in practice it is less common and less clearly required. In contrast the enlisting of the patient and their kith and kin and other community resources underpins much of the thrust toward handling mental disorders in the community rather than in institutional settings. The provision of their own case notes and information regarding treatment modalities to patients would seem a possible way to encourage patient involvement in their own care.

One factor standing in the way of giving case notes to patients hitherto has been the fact that they have been written in pen and ink. This has meant that mistakes made in the tone of the record or clear factual errors cannot be rectified without the recipient being aware that something else was originally in the notes - and without the error remaining there permanently in some form.

In contrast a word processed record could be given to individuals with an explanation that many details will almost certainly be wrong and that they should pinpoint any mistakes and feel free to add further relevant details. This would establish a process that could be expected to lead to further versions of the record which would be likely in most cases to be more accurate and complete than the initial version.

West Aberconwy

The mental health services in Gwynedd are sectorised with Aberconwy being one such sector, having a population of 55,000. It is subdivided into East and West with the Western end having a population of 22,000. West Aberconwy is served by thirteen general practitioners. A mental health team comprised of two consultant psychiatrists, eight community psychiatric nurses, five social workers, a clinical psychologist, an occupational therapist and two junior medical staff covers both West and East Aberconwy flexibly but with one consultant, one junior medical person, three community nurses and two social workers essentially dedicated to the Western end.

As of 1st July, 1990, patients in the West Aberconwy sector of Gwynedd have been getting copies of the letters written to their General Practitioner's (GPs) following out-patient visits, drop-in consultations or domiciliary visits by any team members. Where seen on a number of occasions, a case record or careplan is compiled by the relevant team member, a copy of which the patient also holds. Individuals who are taking neuroleptics or antidepressants on a continuous basis are also given a detailed handout on these drugs - what is known of their mode of action, their benefits and their side effects. These initiatives are used regardless of diagnosis, except in the case of individuals with a clear dementing illness, and they apply to all medical or social data generated on the patient. The various components of this manner of service delivery are outlined in greater detail below.

To date after more than three years of service delivery in this manner, there appears to have been no serious clinical problems generated and no reason not to continue in this manner, although the question of whether these approaches enhance therapeutic efficacy remains to be answered.

Out-patient letters

Ordinarily letters to GPs from out-patient clinics tend to be short giving a diagnostic label and a proposed treatment. In contrast, Aberconwy letters have usually been considerably longer (occasionally running to 3 pages). This betrays the intention, which is that these letters are aimed as much if not more at the patient than their GP.

The letters set out to rehearse what has come up in the out-patient appointment or domiciliary visit for 3 reasons. The first is simply to go over what was said in order to inform the patient, as current research suggests that perhaps only half of what actually gets said is retained by the subject afterwards (Silverman, 1987).

Problems of retention may be particularly prevalent in psychiatry, given that anxiety states will frequently lead to referral and anxiety must be one of the main factors that compromise retention in general medical settings. It is quite common, in my experience, to find that patients have been unable to sleep the night before a clinic visit. This is even true for follow-up visits, when one might expect the level of anxiety to have subsided somewhat. We can therefore add the effects of fatigue on retention to those of anxiety.

A second reason for this approach is to give the patient something they can refer to afterwards or show to their relatives to indicate to them what has been said in order to convince the relatives either that their report of the clinical appointment has been correct or that indeed yes the doctor or mental health team agree that the complaint the individual has is not just simply all in the mind but is in actual fact real (Price and Asch, 1990). Conversely on reading a letter relatives have sometimes felt compelled to come to the clinic or to write to team members to indicate that in their opinion the patient has offered an inaccurate portrayal of the problem.

A final reason for taking this approach is that in psychiatry the traditional wisdom is that a psycho-dynamic (in the broadest sense) interpretation may be curative. After the patient gives their story at some point the "expert" puts it all together and this putting it all together, if correct, should effect clinical change. However, this putting it all together if it is not retained by the patient afterwards is obviously of little use. Putting it in black and white gives the person time to reflect on the issues afterwards - as well as having a 'magic' all of its own.

When the interpretations have been correct or at least helpful, we have had feedback from a number of individuals that they turn to the letters or to the personal file, that a number of them have begun to keep, during times of stress or demoralisation. It appears that having to hand, at such times, a constructive appraisal of the issues they have faced or are facing can be of significant benefit.

A number of other individuals have found themselves prompted to action on receipt of such a letter. Examples have included the confiding in significant others of the details of an abortion or an affair for instance. It is our practice in such cases to refer obliquely rather than explicitly to such matters in cases where it is thought that the material might be sensitive. Thus should the letter inadvertently fall into the wrong hands, confidential material will not be disclosed. However, a clear formulation of the problems and the literal physical bringing of that formulation into the person's home or place of work or whatever, albeit obliquely, appears for some to be a precipitant to action in a way that a simple visit to a clinic rarely is.

This approach confronts a notable feature of clinic attendance behaviour, which appears to be predicated on a tendency on the part of patients referred to a mental health clinic to assume that the psychiatrist or psychologist or whoever can "read their minds". Attenders often appear to assume that there is little need for them to say much - that everything will be transparently obvious. The organisation of the traditional clinic does little to dispel this myth. While veterans of the system at some point become aware of the realities, if such realisation is unmanaged it is all too likely to bring disillusion and cynicism in its wake.

In contrast, actually seeing what the mental health professional has found and seeing that they are only aware of facts that have been discussed in the clinic, that there are no blinding insights from elsewhere or secrets mysteriously conjured out of hats, can be expected to influence subsequent clinic appointments and arguably put the dealings in those appointments on a more realistic basis.

In our practice, patients are told that the purpose for their receiving these letters is for them to either correct the details contained therein and/or to add to the material. This, it is hoped, will engage them more fully in their own care. There are a number of ways in which this can happen other than their simply reporting inaccuracies. One is that anyone else who has contact with the client, whether a community nurse, doctor or social worker then has something to work with. They can go over the material contained in the letter and establish whether the person in question sees this as a reasonable formulation of the problems or indeed has something else to add.

Another way that clients may become engaged is by means of an extension of the concept behind sending these letters - which is to give the patient some work to do in between clinic appointments. A logical extension of this is also to send to the patient various rating scales, of the self-report type, between clinic appointments. For this purpose we have devised a number of our own scales and checklists, including an attitudes to medication questionnaire, a dissociative experiences checklist, a side effects of drugs checklist and others. We also send other checklists for obsessional disorders and standardised self-rating scales for anxiety and depression. Sending the patient checklists or rating scales of this sort permits them to do work in the period between clinic appointments and to bring the results of this work back to subsequent clinics.

There are other forms of work that can be undertaken profitably in this manner - for example paradoxical interventions. Such interventions involve enjoining the patient or their relatives to engage in behaviours that might at first sight seem quite counter-productive such as telling a person who complains of insomnia to try and stay awake all night. Where the focus of therapy is on interactions between family members, paradoxical interventions may become quite complex and accordingly are particularly liable to misinterpretation in face-to-face dialogues in a clinic setting. Couched in black and white and available in the patient's own home for perhaps several weeks between clinic or domiciliary visits, such interpretations would intuitively seem more likely to have an effect.

Finally having received their letter, a number of patients have been quite concerned about what is being held about them in the doctor's file. The reason for their worry concerns the reception staff and what they may have seen. Indeed, one has to wonder whether in clinics in small town or rural settings, with efficient local communication networks, the sending of any letter to a GP might effectively mean that a large part of the community gets to know what is happening. At the very least, the West Aberconwy model would ensure the patient knows what it is that everyone else may know about them.

Pitfalls

There are a number of pitfalls to this approach. One of these is the use of insensitive medical jargon. Where junior medical staff have been engaged in this process, there has been a tendency for them to write to the doctor rather than to the patient - to formulate the patient and leave them pinned and wriggling to a diagnostic schema. One point that can be made is that such formulations, and indeed even less sensitive versions of the same, are finding their way routinely into medical notes as it is, where they are likely to alienate individuals who seek access to their notes in future.

A further issue has been raised by a number of colleagues from other services who have wondered about the problems of full disclosure - how do you tell a person they have schizophrenia? These difficulties highlight what the purpose of the exercise is - which is to do therapy - and that doing therapy in this manner, which involves the committing of often complex constructions to print, may in its own right require some training. Ideally jargon and questions of disclosure should subserve the primary goal which is to move the patient forward. It may be that specific training in this technique will be needed to maximum effectiveness.

If this process is to be taken further, it appears to those of us involved in it that a range of audits will be needed. On a mundane level procedures need to be established such as perhaps informing patients in writing before their clinic appointment that the post-clinic letter will come to them also. Informing them in the clinic has two sets of potential pitfalls associated with it. First, in clinics, particularly when informed during the course of a first attendance, patients are often far too anxious to be able to properly weigh up the pros and cons of receiving such letters. Second, even when told in the clinic that this will be happening, some patients demonstrate one of the reasons for sending the letter to them by failing to remember that they had been told that this would happen; they then rush off to the surgery somewhat guilty or embarrassed at having looked at what they assume is their GP's letter.

Having made these points, however, it should be noted that not only does this practice need to be audited but so also does the more traditional practice of not sending the letter to the patient. It is by no means clear that the traditional practice is harmless.

A second tier of audit would attempt to evaluate the service from the perspectives of both users and professionals and would seek to compare its impact on traditional indices of mental health such as bed usage, drug consumption and rates of suicide with the effects of more traditional approaches.

Multi-disciplinary care-plans

In typical traditional practice, a duty doctor "clerks" the patient in when they first come into the hospital or into an out-patient setting. During subsequent weeks or months what are often skimpy observations are added to the initial clerking. In the case of both in-patients and out-patients, quite separately to this, nurses will hold a record of nursing observations on the patient. There may even be two sets of nursing observations, one the record of in-patient observations and the other held by community nurses. In all cases, however, observations are simply added on to an initial history. For in-patients, at the point of discharge, a discharge summary goes to the general practitioner. This discharge summary and both the medical and nursing notes in all instances inadequately reflect the amount of knowledge about the individual in care that has been garnered during the course of treatment. And more importantly, the form in which this knowledge is held does not permit constructive access for any user be they mental health worker, GP or patient.

Access by patients to such notes is furthermore generally seen as problematic. One reason for this as noted above has probably been simply the fact that notes hitherto have been compiled in pen and ink and have not been readily changeable as a consequence. If notes/careplans are work-processed, an entirely different prospect emerges. Uncertainties, sensitive material and the range of attitudes members of the team have had about individuals can be included secure in the knowledge that, if the recipient takes exception, details can be changed or that "negotiations" can be commenced about what are, ipso facto, quite likely to be key issues.

What happens in Aberconwy in practice is that when the patient first comes into contact with the services a detailed history is taken in the usual manner. This, however, is word processed rather than just simply written or typed. It is, furthermore, composed in the knowledge that it will subsequently be handed to the patient and possibly also to their next of kin, shortly after entry into treatment, whether out-patient or in-patient.

The purpose of this is three fold. One is to inform the patient about the details and opinions that are held on their files about their case. Quite apart from the traditional patient curiosity about what their medical notes might contain, there is the problem noted above that in psychiatry patients often have quite unrealistic ideas of just what information might be held on them.

The second function is to collect data. There are two ways in which this can happen. The first is that the patient on reading the material may be able to inform us that certain data are wrong - for instance, we have been told that spouses we have recorded as having died several years previously are in actual fact alive and well. Such errors can then be corrected. The more important aspect, however, is that it will become clear from a first draft of the careplan on a particular patient that our information is quite incomplete.

The advantage of a word processed version of the casenotes is that a standard outline (see appendix) can be handed to the patient into which the data that has already been gathered on them has been slotted. In such an outline important areas that need filling will initially be blank. The patient and their next of kin are encouraged to provide the further data that is needed as regards personal background, social circumstances, attitudes towards treatment, fears about the illness and about therapists, etc.

As can be seen from our outline careplan (see appendix), there is an anthropological turn to the information we are seeking. In addition to the usual headings under which medical notes are collected, we have included some extra patient-centred categories, drawn from the work of Arthur Kleinman on the anthropology of chronic illness (Kleinman, 1988). These include the sections on presenting problem, personal diagnosis, effects of treatment and potential pitfalls (see appendix).

There have been two reasons for including these categories. One has been the belief that in psychiatry and in particular in chronic conditions the patient's view of the problem is often more important than the therapist's. This form of the record therefore will act as much as anything else as a reminder to the mental health worker of areas they may not have explored.

A second reason is that it was hoped that the inclusion of categories in the case record clearly labelled as categories constructed for the purpose of eliciting the patient's own observations regarding the cause of their illness, their understanding of that illness and attitudes towards treatment would promote the more general process of obtaining patient input to their own record - to ensure accuracy and to augment data collection.

A third point is that a careplan should ideally pull together the different perceptions of the medical, psychological, social work and nursing staff. All should be able to contribute to the same careplan. If they were, this would provide a certain consistency of therapeutic input. All too often individuals who come into the mental health services find themselves being confronted with one view of what is wrong with them by a clinical psychologist, a different view by social workers, several other views by the nursing staff and yet further views by the medical staff with perhaps the consultant and junior medical staff both having different views. This can at best be confusing and risks being harmful. A single multidisciplinary record, to which the patient has access has the potential to improve this state of affairs. It also potentially provides the patient with a tool to confront members of staff who might be proposing alternative viewpoints - a method perhaps to control "rogue" staff, be they medical, nursing, psychological or social workers.

Indeed a logical extension of this practice would be to have clients construct their own care plans, according to the agreed framework, with the therapists' role being to review it and amending details or adding further details by negotiation. This has been done in a small number of cases - the numbers at present are restricted more by difficulties in gaining access to the requisite technology than by anything else.

Finally, the same careplan is given to the general practitioner, for example in the form of a discharge summary in the case of individuals who have been in-patients. The GP is encouraged to contribute to it on the basis of their knowledge of the patient in their social network. This potentially provides a more formal channel for interaction between the primary health team and specialised services than is usually available.

It is envisaged that this process of setting up a careplan will happen for all patients admitted to hospital and for all individuals seen on three or more occasions. This means that a large number of out-patients will in due course have careplans also.

A pilot study on this kind of shared careplan has been carried out in London (Essex et al., 1990). In this study patients liked seeing what had been written about them and the idea of holding their own record was welcomed although there were some anxieties expressed about having their names and diagnoses recorded. In the view of the researchers in this study the main obstacle to adopting this approach more regularly lay in the attitude of doctors, nurses and managers. However, Essex et al., (1990) only included selected patients and they did not give patients access to all the information about them on which the careplan was based.

Consensus statements

In addition to providing the patient with a personalised careplan, the Aberconwy team has been working of consensus statements on the various drug or non-drug therapies and the latest thinking on the key clinical features of psychiatric disorders, such as delusions, hallucinations, obsessions, etc.

There are three reasons for doing this. The first is the process of producing consensus statements. To be useful a statement about neuroleptics, for example, cannot just be the views of the medical consultant. Such statements need to be the view of the team who will be treating the patient. That is the team needs to sit down and work out exactly what they think neuroleptics do, list their side-effects, etc.

Such a consensus view may not actually represent the views of any one individual but is a view that the team is happy to work with for a specified period of time, be it three months, six months or a year, after which ideally the various consensus statements should be evaluated in terms of consistency with current knowledge and the degree to which they meet the needs that are thrown up by clinical practice. As a result of one such recent evaluation, our current set of statements are being rewritten by service users.

The second reason for such statements is to inform patients. All too often in clinical practice what happens is that patients are told to "take the pills". They are rarely, if ever, told much about the pills. It is left to their own devices if they wish to seek out further information about the various pills, much of which, drawn from sources such as popular magazines, may be harmful. And a great number of individuals simply suffer the side-effects often unaware that the side-effects are side-effects.

For example, a patient who develops akathisia on neuroleptics often attributes the restless, nervous feelings they have to a worsening of their own nervous problems rather than to a drug-induced side-effect (Healy, 1993). It is not uncommon, for example, to have patients become upset in clinic at the idea of their medication being halted, who, when the matter is pursued further, indicate that it is the anticholinergic antidote that they are on that they would be reluctant to lose rather than the major tranquilliser. Such a state of affairs is potentially counter-therapeutic.

The purpose of the handout on neuroleptics, therefore, by including the range of side-effects that the drugs can produce is to inform the patient of what the drugs do and do not do and of the various problems they may cause. The object of the exercise is to enlist the patient as a responsible co-therapist, where possible. It is our belief that this can only be done in so far as the patient has as complete an access to the available information as is possible.

The third reason for consensus statements is to collect data. Very often we simply do not know the full range of side-effects that these drugs may produce or the full extent to which the use of these drugs may interfere with a person's life. More importantly we really have very little clue, particularly in the case of the neuroleptics, about what it is that these drugs do that is good and useful. The purpose of the exercise, therefore, in this case is to try and elicit from the patient further information about what these drugs usefully do for them.

This function of consensus statements would seem best served by systematic research through user groups. This could be done in a number of different ways. One way would be to give patients the handouts and an accompanying diary to record whether they used the handout or not. If they did, then the question is whether it helped them usefully on the particular point or problem that they had, recording at the actual time, if possible, any further observations they might have to add to the core statement.

Another method of collecting the data would be to bring a group of handout users together, to discuss, as a group, the usefulness or otherwise of the handouts. With the help of others who may have glimmers of what they are trying to articulate, individuals struggling to account for the effects of drugs on them may find themselves able to come to a fuller and, for our purposes, a much more useful articulation of the issues involved.

Even before getting to such a structured format, the information collected from users in response to being given these handouts has proved illuminating. In the case of the handout on neuroleptics, for example, it was hoped that we would be able to collect information on how individuals find these drugs useful in their daily life - there is a great dearth of client centred information on this. We have been relatively successful in this, gaining some memorable descriptions such as the following: a patient described how while on neuroleptics he felt as though he was living in a tunnel with no light at the end of it but a tunnel which was wide and had cushioned sides - off the drugs light appeared at the end of the tunnel but the sides closed in and sharp and painful edges protruded from them. More generally, the positive effects of neuroleptics have been described in terms of diminishing preoccupation or taking the edge off intrusive worries or ideas.

As regards side effects we have had patients report on a great number of side effects that they have been having which were not detailed in the original handouts. These include, in the case of neuroleptics for example, drinking vast amounts of tea and coffee while on these drugs and in particular a neuroleptic withdrawal syndrome that involves nightmares, stiffness and other features. This latter is not well described in the literature. In the case of antidepressants we have become more aware of depersonalisation and derealisation effects as well as an increased frequency of myoclonic jerks and other unusual, rarely noted side effects.

The reports we have had from patients have also led to appreciation of some finer details of neuroleptic pharmacology. A number of patients have said that their sleep quality is much better off neuroleptics than on neuroleptics. This is of interest given the general impression that neuroleptics are in some way sedative and a widespread use of neuroleptics in in-patient settings is for sedative purposes. However, patient perceptions have proved accurate on this point - it is now clear that some neuroleptics, while being sedative at some doses, may be stimulant at others and that sleep quality may indeed be poor on them (a fact employed by Lundbeck in their marketing of flupenthixol as an antidepressant neuroleptic - see Healy, 1993).

There is a further important aspect to collecting this kind of information, in that patient reports on side-effects tend to give a much better impression of the practical problems of taking neuroleptics than is gained from the checklist of adverse events that focus part of the typical clinical trial of a new drug. For example, one individual reported to us having to buy a bra two sizes larger than usual for her; of finding herself becoming amenorrhoeic on neuroleptics and, assuming she was infertile as a consequence, engaging in unprotected sexual activity (that fortunately did not lead to pregnancy but which could easily have done so because the lack of menses caused by a neuroleptic is no safeguard against conception). This patient also had a side-effect, common to many subjects on neuroleptics, of putting on a considerable amount of weight; she then had the experience of being told by her GP and others that she was fat and that she should try hard to lose weight, which produced problems in that it is often not possible to lose weight easily while on neuroleptics. Unaware that the weight gain could be caused by the drugs, she had become guilty and demoralised.

A further aspect to the handouts is that patients read extensively on the subject of their illnesses and treatments as it is. They may only be reading magazines or they may progress to taking books from the library or buying one of the increasing range of self-help books for nerves, popular guides to drug consumption or commentaries on the use of psychotropic drugs in clinical practice (viz Gorman, 1989; Breggin, 1993; Lacey, 1992; and the British National Formulary to which a great number of patients appear to have access). As a general principle, indeed it would probably be wise to assume that most patients are engaged in finding out about their illness or their treatments.

In many cases it is probable that unless there is a very clear and explicit message from the mental health team, in black and white, the message from popular magazines or from television programmes is likely to outweigh anything that comes from the clinic. The best way to counter-balance this is to provide explicit information that can be compared with information obtained from elsewhere and to invite the patient to bring back any significant discrepancies they find to the clinic and ask for a resolution.

Overview and evaluation?

To some extent, the method of service delivery outlined here simply avails of the opportunities thrown up by the recent development of word processing packages. Previously, the kind of transformations of formulations outlined above were prohibitively cumbersome - a simple serial record of information was all that was practicable.

The value put on a system such as this will depend on the primary therapeutic goals of any mental health professionals involved in its use. Within the Aberconwy team the dominant value professed is one of fostering competence - of empowering the patient. While one cannot say of this system that it will unambiguously foster competence - information overload may damage some individuals - it would seam probable that for most individuals the system will at the very least not be as disempowering as traditional systems are.

The ways in which careplans and letters can be used to empower patients were noted above. Others have included the use of such materials on the part of patients to convey information to their family that was felt to be too sensitive to convey in face-to-face interaction. Patients have for example left careplans lying around at home expecting them to be read by others who would thereby find out about suspected child abuse. A further patient on acquiring his case history laid out in systematic form was struck by the drama of his story and has embarked on an attempt to fictionalise it.

The mode of operating here aims at enlisting patients as co-therapists in the management of their own disorders. This a project somewhat different to those that arise from the current emphasis on fostering user involvement in the design and management of mental health services. It is not impossible that user involvement in a therapeutic sense could coincide with a paternalistic approach to service development but in practice this seems unlikely. This could be assessed by systematically collecting patients' observations of the care delivery systems they encounter at the same time that their views on their condition and its treatment are being collected.

In practice family views have not been spontaneously forthcoming to date. In part this must stem from the fact that where these views are most likely to be of interest, it will be because the family are part of the problem. Short of them engaging the family in therapy, it may not be possible to access these views with any degree of frequency.

It has also been difficult to engage general practitioners in the system. At present work is underway to establish whether letters and careplans are used by patients or by GPs in their mutual encounters. A number of GPs have been faced on call with patients unknown to them who have quoted directly from clinic letters as to what their problems are and what needs to be done. It is not clear to what extent this is happening and whether it is helpful.

One might indeed question how useful or indeed therapeutic it would be to have 100% GP compliance with the system. There may be as yet unexplored dangers in understanding the patient too well or in the extreme dominance of one type of understanding.

There are further problems in that the ideal GP input would require psychotherapeutic skills of the GP of a high order as well as an ability to commit these to print - something that trainee psychiatric staff have difficulty with.

Finally, to function properly, systems such as this would need to be in place county-wide as a great deal of information is generated on patients during in-patient periods in hospital or hostels. If processing capacity is only based in community mental health teams, a great deal of this information will be effectively lost or else the burden of recording basic personal information - which must be recorded for an episode of in-patient care - will fall entirely on the CMHT. At present, in Aberconwy, just this difficulty is inhibiting fuller implementation of this approach.

The developments described above mark a change from a paternalistic to a participative service orientation. This involves taking a very different attitude towards the public and is founded on a willingness to take consumer views seriously, encouraging the expression of views and responding constructively to them (Deakin and Wright, 1990). Clarke and Steward, (1986) described this as representing a change in emphasis from services to the public to services for the public. They suggest that this new orientation involves closeness to the public, listening to the public, seeking out views, suggestions and complaints from the public point of view, acknowledging the public's right to know, emphasising service quality and using the public as a test of that quality.

Defining the proper degree of user or public participation in health care is difficult, given the requirement for consumer protection at one end of the spectrum and citizen or community action of a radical nature at the other (Maxwell and Weaver, 1984). Nevertheless, Potter (1988), for example, argues that participation comes down to user or citizen empowerment, implying power sharing if not partnership between users and providers of services. Power-sharing however, is multi-dimensional, involving questions such as: what value do public service managers and procurers put on user involvement? to what extent are public services prepared to accept users as judges? and how far is it the intention to redress the imbalance of power that has existed between providers and users? In psychiatric practice there is a further dimension in that user empowerment may in its own right be therapeutic.

An analysis of user involvement developments framed in this way has the potential to elucidate the respective strengths of any criteria proposed as vital elements of process. For example, a pilot study of shared care records for people with mental illness showed that patients found them very acceptable and they were enthusiastic about their use (Essex, Doig and Renshaw, 1990). They liked seeing what had been written about them and the idea of holding their own records was welcomed, though there were some anxieties expressed about having the individual's name, address and diagnosis recorded. The main obstacles to the approach were seen as the attitudes, perceptions and fears of doctors, nurses and managers. This research, however, has to be treated cautiously because the questionnaires used were administered by members of the psychiatric team rather than by an observer with no vested interests in treatment plans.

In similar vein a recent account of patients' reactions to letters from psychiatric consultants after out-patient consultations (Price and Asch, 1990) indicated a number of key benefits to patients. The findings indicated that patients on the whole liked receiving the letters and none were hostile or upset by the experience. For some there were suggestions that improvements in self-esteem were discernible and for others it was advantageous to have an account which acted as an aide-memoire and which could be shown to sceptical relatives. However, in contrast to the practice within West Aberconwy, only a small proportion of those patients eligible to participate in the initiative did so, and of those that did most were suffering from depressive, anxiety or psychosomatic disorders.

It has long been acknowledged that passive reception of drugs from harried or preoccupied professionals does little to prepare to teach patients to use medication autonomously. Indeed studies indicate that between 25% and 94% of psychiatric patients who attend out-patient clinics fail to take their medication as prescribed (Baeklund and Lundwall, 1975, Eisenthal et al., 1979). Equally there are accounts showing that more relaxed and discursive approaches with chronic schizophrenic patients, and the involvement of their informal carers, can raise significantly compliance with drug treatments (Liberman and Davis, 1975). Importantly this appeared to be linked to a reduction in the use of in-patient and day hospital facilities. Whether this potential holds for consensus statements, which represent a more systematic method for conveying important data about drugs to patients, appears to be worth investigating.

In terms of practices within Aberconwy, above and beyond any audit of the practical operational details of the system, there is clearly a need for research on what is being done that would go beyond simple assessments of patient/user satisfaction - for research which describes user involvement strategies in practice, which explicates the benefits from the perspective of users and providers, and which demonstrates the nature of any system gains in terms of the better use of resources.

In terms of benefits to users and professionals there is a need to interview users to define what they have found of value in the respective user involvement strategies adopted by the team, focusing on accounts of how newly referred and patients previously treated elsewhere experience the mental health services. How individuals make sense of strategies that have been designed to help them is of central concern.

Interviews with users can be expected to be helpful in flagging up indicators of intermediate output. For example, users can be questioned about treatment and service in terms of health quality criteria (Maxwell, 1984). Potentially, these would provide an indication of the accessibility, acceptability, flexibility, reliability, sufficiency and co-ordination of services from the point of view of the user. While not providing answers to questions about clinical improvement or well-being, they may well be predictive in this regard. Ideally the same individuals would be followed up after six months or a year, to establish whether their experiences have changed. By this time it is likely that they would have become more familiar with the idea of both the care plans and the consensus statements so their expectations may have changed too.

Since carers can play vital support roles in assisting treatment compliance, it would be of interest to take account of their views of what has been done to inform and involve them in case management terms. It should also be possible to use their accounts as a means of validating the views expressed by users and, as necessary, force into the open any contradictions between them, hopefully in a manner that can be explained.

It would be useful also to interview GPs in the area about the written responses they receive following referrals. The form and content of these letters requires some appraisal from the perspective of GPs if they are to be properly informed about the best treatment for individuals, particularly as in these days of community care they are a key channel through which users are to be helped and treated.

It would also be critical to make some attempt to appraise the views of community mental health team members as to what benefits individual members derive for their own professional practice from investing in these activities. It is not clear that there has ever been any work of this kind reported.

In addition to appraising the reported experiences of individuals about user involvement, which may say more about the perceptions and subjective impressions of those concerned than about what actually takes place, if sense is to be made of such accounts, it would be important to invest some research time into recording exactly how user involvement strategies are put in place, through observation of case management meetings and other team activities. It can be expected that shared goals and approaches to work, attitudes of team leaders or co-ordinators, local work organisation, specialist division of labour, and procedural issues relating to workload management and needs assessment would play a significant part in determining the extent to which user involvement strategies would be put into practice (Crosbie and Vickery, 1989).

As regards to system impacts it would be desirable to know whether the investment of staff time in user involvement of this type is helpful in maintaining treatment compliance. Indicators could be derived from an analysis of case plans, comparing these with user and carer accounts obtained by interview and comparing compliance levels with other teams in Gwynedd using different approaches. There are suggestions that interventions of the kind reflected by the team's development work may well lead to reductions in hospital bed use and this in turn could be monitored.

A third level at which system impacts could be gauged is through the account of the team members themselves. There would be no point in continuing with user involvement developments if teams were of the view that these were not serving some kind of therapeutic purpose for users, or if they were making such demands on staff that clinical work was being impaired. This can be problematical where professionals embrace development work in their clinical practice (Wiston and Wray, 1987).

Acknowledgements

The ideas expressed above owe a great deal to discussions with Barry Broadmeadow, Pat Corns, Bill Creaney, Mary Davies, Louise Doughty,

Gordon Grant, John Harlow, Jane Hollywood, Robin Holden, Jean Hughes, Niall Maclean, Ian Murry, Alison Pearson, Colin Peters, Julia Pook, Eleri Price, Adrian Pugh, Ian Rickard, Rebecca Sykes, Brian Williams and Hilary Yeadon.

Appendix

Casenote outline

A. Personal

   1. General
        1) Date of birth
        2) Address and telephone number(s)
        3) Status
        4) Children
        5) Next of kin
        6) Occupation
        7) National health number

   2. Significant personal details

        1) Place in family
        2) Parents and their occupations
        3) Childhood
        4) Emotional tone of home
        5) Health in childhood
        6) School career - academic & social
        7) Work record
        8) Relationships

   3. Personality and values

        1) Social network
        2) Leisure activities
        3) Predominant mood
        4) Character
        5) Beliefs and values

   4. Social circumstances

        1) Marriage
        2) Children
        3) Current employment
        4) Financial
        5) Housing
        6) Legal

5. Medical history

   a. General medical

      1) respiratory
      2) Cardiac
      3) Abdominal
      4) Renal
      5) Genital
      6) Skeletal
      7) Eyes/ENT
      8) Skin
      9) Operations
      10) X-Rays
      11) Lab tests

   b. Psychological

      1) Dates in/out patient treatment
      2) Details of therapists
      3) Problem
      4) Diagnosis
      5) Treatment

   c. Family medical and mental health history

      1) Father
      2) Mother
      3) Siblings
      4) Spouse
      5) Children

   d. Medication history

      1) Prescribed
      2) Over the counter
      3) Alcohol
      4) Smoking
      5) Other substances

   e. Other therapies

      1) Psychological
      2) Alternative

B.	Case

1.	Presenting problem

1)	Initial view
2)	Initial agreed view
3)	Current view

2.	Background to problem

3.	Concurrent symptoms

1)	Anxiety - physical/mental
2)	Obsessions
3)	Phobias
4)	Traumatic memories
5)	Health concerns
6)	Mood
7)	Memory
8)	Thinking
9)	Hallucinations
10)	Beliefs

4.	Personal diagnosis

1)	Diagnosis
2)	Cause
3)	Why it is a problem now
4)	Effect on life
5)	What I fear most about this illness
Going crazy
Being committed
Suicide
Effects of drugs
Passing it on to my children
Never getting back to normal

5.	Professional diagnosis

1)	Formulation
2)	Code
3)	Cause
4)	Why it is a problem now

6. Treatment history

      1) Treatment history
      2) Effects of treatment - personal view
      3) Effects of treatment - professional view

7. Action plan

      1) Drugs
      2) Physical viz exercise
      3) Avoid viz alcohol

      4) Behaviour therapy
      5) Cognitive therapy
      6) Counselling
      7) Analytic therapy
      8) Family therapy

      9) Employment
      10) Accommodation
      11) Finances

      12) Who is involved
               Subject
               Team Member
               Others
      13) Starting date
      14) Ending date

      15) Potential pitfalls
               personal view
               professional view

8. Family view of problem

9. GP's view of problem

References

Baeklund, F. and Lundwall, L. (1975) 'Dropping out of treatment : a critical review', *Psychological Bulletin* no. 82, 738-783.

Breggin, P. (1993) *Toxic Psychiatry,* Fontana Press, London.

Bursztajn, H.J., Feinbloom, R.I., Hamm, R.M. and Brodsky, A. (1990) *Medical Choices. Medical Chances,* Routledge, London.

Clarke, M. and Steward, J. (1986) *The Public Service Orientation : Developing the Approach*, Luton, Local Goverment Training Board.

Corrigan, P., Liberman R. and Engel, J. (1990), 'From noncompliance to collaboration in the treament of Schizophrenia', *Hospital and Community Psychiatry* no. 41, 1203-1211.

Crosbie, D. and Vickery A. (1989) *Community based schemes in area offices : report to the Department of Health,* National Institute for Social Work, London.

Deakin, N. and Wright, A. (1990) *Consuming Public Services,* Routledge, London.

Eisenthal, S., Emery R. and Lazare, A. (1979) 'Adherence and the negotiated approach to patienthood', *Archives of General Psychiatry* no. 36, 393-398.

Essex, B., Doig R. and Renshaw J. (1990) 'Pilot study of records of shared care for people with mental illnesses', *British Medical Journal,* no. 300, 1442-1446.

Gorman, J. (1989) *The Essential Guide to Psychiatic Drugs,* St Martin's Press, New York.

Healy, D. (1993) *Psychiatric Drugs Explained,* Wolfe Medical Publishers, London.

Kleinman, A. (1988) *The Illness Narratives,* Basic Books, New York.

Lacey, R. (1992) *The Mind Guide to Psychiatric Drugs,* Edbury Press, London.

Liberman, R. and Davis, J. (1975) 'Drugs and behaviour analysis', *Progress in Behaviour Modification,* no.1, 307-330.

Maxwell, R. (1984) 'Quality assessment in health,' *British Medical Journal,* no. 288.

Maxwell, R. and Weaver, N. (1984) 'Public participation in health : Towards a clearer view', King Edward's Hospital Fund for London.

Potter, J. (1988) 'Consumerism and the public sector : how well does the coat fit? *Public Administration,* no. 66, 149-164.

Price, J.S. and Asch R. (1990) 'Writing to the Patient', *Psychiatric Bulletin,* July, 8. 467-469.

Silverman, D. (1987) *Communication and Medical Practice,* Sage Publications, London.

Wiston, G. and Wray, K. (1987) 'Community mental handicap teams: service delivery and service development: The Nottinghamshire approach' in Grant, C., Humphreys S. and McGrath, M. (eds) *CMHTs Theory and Practice,* British Insitute of Mental Handicap, Kidderminster.

231

10 Users' views of community mental health care

Brian Williams

Summary

This chapter is based on an ongoing qualitative study of users' views of mental health services. In depth interviews were conducted with long term users with inpatient experience and new referrals to community mental health services. Criticisms held by those with past inpatient experience included a general lack of respect, frequent re-diagnoses, the removal of their ability to complain by viewing complaints as 'symptoms', and a sense of powerlessness resulting in fear.

Most current methods of collating user opinion provide data at a descriptive level which fails to explain why users have the criticisms they do. Users' views of community services are explored and a case study used to demonstrate the need for further research into the way in which users evaluate community mental health services. New referrals to such services have a host of beliefs about psychiatrists and the nature of mental disorders. These beliefs and concerns interact with the reality of service provision to produce disillusionment or satisfaction. The outcome may include criticisms regarding waiting times, privacy, health professionals' manner and the impersonal nature of the service. Only by listening to users' views and understanding their origin can community services be developed which, in twenty years time, will not face the same criticisms users currently make about inpatient care.

Introduction

Users' opinions matter. This has increasingly been the conclusion of government, the public and mental health professionals (HMSO, 1984; HMSO, 1989). It has, however, been a long time in coming and for many of those service users who believe they have been treated badly the

233

practical outworking of such political beliefs may not be seen for some time. Legislation may be introduced over night while role or power related changes may take years, if not generations.

Considering the prominence given to shifting the balance of mental health care towards the community, it is surprising how little we know of service users' views. There has been much public, political and academic debate over community care policy with user groups playing their part in each sphere. However, too often it is asked 'what do service users think of this or that issue?' when instead the question should be 'what issues are important to service users?'. Putting users at the centre of service provision means allowing them to set the agenda of what is and what is not important or problematic rather than giving their opinions on predetermined issues. Consumerism, accountability and democratisation mean more than asking users what they think of the food; it concerns empowerment which must mean listening to the voice users have always had but which is often ignored because they are 'mentally ill'.

This paper is not concerned with comparing users' perspectives of hospital and community services in terms of their availability, accessibility and convenience. To do so would be to paternalistically set the users' agenda of importance. Rather, it takes users' accounts of their experience of mental health care, draws out those issues which are important to them, and questions whether the move towards community based care provides a solution. Most of the quotes in this chapter necessarily contain complaints about the status quo; however, this does not mean that the experience of all users is negative. During the course of the interviews many complimentary remarks were made concerning the staff, their commitment and the service as a whole.

I begin with a brief look at some historical accounts of users' views, and then move on to a number of interviews with those with more recent experience. As we shall see it is curious how some issues have remained unchanged.

A historical legacy

Latent political structures govern the way in which the history of a time is recorded. Consequently, the lack of accounts of service users' experiences in the eighteenth and nineteenth centuries tells its own story. On the whole the voice of the 'insane' was not considered important. In contemporary debate the explanation for the lack of importance attached to patients' views is in terms of the traditional passive patient sick role. However, such an explanation might not be applicable to a time when the medical profession was still trying to claim a monopoly of cure over mental disorder (Scull, 1989, p.127) and when there was much public disillusion with their attempts (Shyrock, 1979). The lack of credibility given to users' views more likely stemmed from the way in which 'madness' was perceived and the social position of the individual concerned.

The nature of 'madness' In the eighteenth and nineteenth centuries considerable stigma was attached to having a member of one's family certified. Consequently, those who were certified were generally those considered too 'difficult' or 'embarrassing' to be cared for at home. To be certified was to be seen as seriously deviant (Scull, 1989, p.124) implying a detachment from normality which rendered one's opinions invalid; after all the very process of certification legally justified the usurping of an individual's basic rights.

For some health professionals at least, certification meant that the opinions of service users must be invalid. This is apparent in a report of a speech given by Hayes Newington to the Medico-Psychological Association in July, 1886.

> taking patients themselves, the acute maniac did not care where he was, the melancholic would be miserable anywhere, and it was principally the 'moral insanity' cases which made the most noise from the patient's point of view, and they were just the people in asylums whose opinions should be considered the least. (Hayes Newington, 1886, p.301)

It can be seen that the perceived nature of mental disorder contributed greatly to the undermining of user opinion; to be certified was to be regarded as one who does not have the ability to make sensible and reasonable comments on care received (Scull, 1989, p.86). Eighteenth century literature on insanity stressed;

> an almost exclusive emphasis on disturbances of the reason, or the higher intellectual faculties of man. Insanity was conceived as a derangement of those very faculties which were widely assumed to be universal to man; as a matter of fact, we sometimes find in the literature the presumed absence in animals of any condition analogous to insanity taken as proof that man's highest psychological function results from some principle totally lacking in other animals, that is the soul. (Scull, 1989, p.88)

William Tuke, the originator of moral treatment, however, argued for an analogy between the judicious treatment of children and that of insane persons; this led to a form of care which sought to re-educate patients and teach them to reassert their powers of self control. This also entailed a greater level of respect for users' views (De La Rive, 1798; Smith, 1814). As Scull has commented:

> This approach involved treating the patient as much in the manner of a rational being, as the state of mind will possibly allow, rather than using motives of fear as a way of managing the patient. Far from harshness being necessary to avoid violent outbreaks among the inmates, it tended only to produce them. (Scull, 1989, p.29-30)

Social position Financial security effectively meant that some rights and autonomy could be retained and one's opinions respected by becoming a 'customer' rather than a 'patient'. A number of private asylums existed for the middle and upper classes, the most notable of these being Ticehurst in Kent. To market themselves effectively to private patients the quality of care had to be superior to that of public asylums; this necessarily included a degree of respect for each patient and a recognition of their basic human dignity despite any mental condition. Respect shown to the user probably stemmed from a desire to retain business and not from a belief in the inherent value of users' opinions (Hayes Newington, 1886).

Despite mixed motives it is generally believed that private asylums did provide a better service.

> Attendants at Ticehurst were expected to treat patients with the respect normally accorded by servants to members of a superior class. One attendant was dismissed 'for not saluting the ladies as provided in our regulations'. In 1881, the commissioners commented that 'the fact that this is a private asylum, is, as far as possible, veiled by the comfort and elegancies of the house and furniture.' The case-notes on a female patient called Lucy Bing Tinne record that she: 'Does not appear to recognise the ladies about her are insane, looks upon this building as an hotel (MacKenzie, 1985, p.166).

Users' issues

The written history of psychiatric institutions tends to be the history of psychiatric treatment rather than the experience of service users. The perspective we are interested in is that of the patient and it is indicative of the regard for service users at the time that such a historical perspective is difficult to identify.

Service users' accounts are limited to court records and biographies - both more the domain of the upper and middle classes than the typical working person. The issues raised in such documents cannot be considered as representative of all service users; nevertheless, they remain important.

Wrongful confinement

Wrongful confinements could be seen as falling into two categories: those arising from an inappropriate classification of an individual due to the blurring of insanity and eccentricities in one's character; and secondly, those where genuine conspiracies had taken place.

An example of the former is the case of Louisa Nottidge (Scull, 1989) who was certified on the basis of her involvement with a small religious cult. The case of William Belcher is of the conspiracy sort (Porter, 1987). Locked up in a private asylum in Hackney from 1778 to 1795 Belcher claims that he was perfectly sane when certified by a jury which had never met him. The reason for this, he claimed, was to facilitate the seizure of his estates. This was certainly not an isolated incident as the experiences of Samuel Bruckshaw and Walter Marshall testify (Porter, 1987; MacKenzie, 1985).

Lack of respect

Madness was perceived as removing an important element of one's humanity. It is inevitable, therefore, that this belief sometimes resulted in disrespectful behaviour. However, it also manifested itself in two other areas; firstly, in the lack of information given to patients, and secondly, in the way in which users' words and actions were viewed as products of their illness.

Lack of information In January 1832 John Perceval was admitted to Brislington Asylum run by Dr Edward Long Fox, a quaker. After eventually being moved on to the more up market 'Ticehurst' Perceval recovered and wrote about his experience. While admitting that for a time he was insane, he argues that this was exacerbated while in the asylum by the treatment regimes and the basic lack of respect afforded him. Perceval makes the following comments:

> I was never told such and such things we are going to do; we think it advisable to administer such and such medicine, in this or that manner; I was never asked, Do you want anything? do you wish for, prefer anything? have you any objection to this or that? Overall I was no longer a free agent, but under the control of beings superiorly enlightened (Mackenzie, 1985, p.182).

It is clear that the behaviour of the staff and Perceval's reaction both stem from their own perceptions of 'madness'. On the staff's behalf this originated in a conviction that he had lost his ability to reason and understand any information given to him. Perceval's view of insanity, however, judged by firsthand experience, was that it involved a 'complex interweaving of the imbecile and perverse with the rational and willing'. In his experience 'the residues of reason were never given the support they needed'.

The interpretation of complaints The validity ascribed to one's views may be found in the way in which one's opinions or behaviour are interpreted. For Perceval little could be done it seemed without it being regarded as a symptom of madness.

> They (servants) were disrespectful, rude and entirely lacking in true deference... Patients of a superior rank such as himself were, of course, honour-bound to display a gallant resentment to this mockery, insult and oppression, but such displays of English spirit were taken in turn as the signs of mania. (MacKenzie, 1985, p.183)

Porter makes the following comment on the regime:

> It was intrinsically so mad and maddening that any patient with normal healthy impulses would indeed be driven mad by it. Yet the system also demanded the acquiescence and compliance of the mad themselves. The inmate who protested against the order of the asylum was thought to be mad, indeed suspect, suffering from 'suspicion' which constituted part of his delusions... if he resists the treatment, he is then a madman (MacKenzie, 1985, p.185).

In an earlier quote Hayes Newington commented that 'the acute melancholic would be miserable anywhere' (Hayes Newington, 1886); on such a basis any complaint a melancholic did make would be seen as further proof of their illness. If one's 'normal' responses to inappropriate treatment are interpreted as further evidence of one's illness there is little an individual can say or do to remedy the situation. The powerlessness of the service user in such a scenario is frightening.

Disempowerment

The preceding two issues indicate that disempowerment was the major underlying problem service users faced. Food, accommodation, daily regime, treatment plans and medication types can only ever be responsive to user opinion when that opinion has some inherent value and power. This sense of powerlessness was rooted in the perceived nature of madness at the time (Scull, 1989). Such perceptions have changed, safeguards against wrongful confinement have increased, and users consulted on a variety of issues; but have the fundamental issues of importance to inpatients and those using community based services really changed? Furthermore, are the current changes towards community care and increased consumerism in health services really addressing all the major concerns of users?

Contemporary mental health care

Accessing users' views of eighteenth and nineteenth century psychiatric care is a relatively inaccurate affair. As mentioned earlier we are reliant upon incidental reports since no formal method of collating user opinion existed. In contemporary psychiatric health care we believe we are in the process of putting such methods in place. While the vast majority of methodologies currently take the form of patient satisfaction surveys there are increasing doubts as to their validity and their ability to accurately embody users' views (Fitzpatrick and Hopkins, 1983; Williams, 1994). This is an important point and worth considering briefly.

Current methods for collating user opinion range in scale and sophistication from the ad hoc study which, in practical terms, is little more than a token gesture to consumerism, through to the highly financed CASPE system (Clinical Accountability, Service Planning and Evaluation) which includes service reorientation as an integral element. Whether either can provide an accurate portrait of service users' views is debatable. There are a number of reasons for this.

Calnan (1988a) and Locker & Dunt (1978) have noted that while questions asked in surveys tend to point to high levels of 'satisfaction', service users often display a more critical nature when given the opportunity, through more open ended questions, to express themselves in their own terms. Consequently, quantitatively measured satisfaction tends to be high (Lebow, 1983) while qualitative reports reveal greater levels of disquiet (Calnan, 1988a; Gabe and Lipshitz-Phillips, 1984).

A further concern is that many quantitative methodologies concentrate on asking service users their opinions of specific aspects of care whether they be food, general hotel facilities, waiting times or technical treatment. Such information is useful and valid but only consists of independent snippets of information which may or may not be related by some wider concern. Addressing satisfaction survey results alone may be to deal with symptoms of an underlying issue rather than the issue itself.

From the jigsaw that makes up the user's overall perspective we may know what ten or fifteen individual pieces look like but have no idea of the overall picture itself nor how the pieces we do have relate to one another. This is the crux issue: users' views do not consist of thirty or forty independent one word replies to preset questions. Users' views embody a complex web of beliefs and concerns, some held tentatively and others zealously, but each with its own rationale and justification available to the researcher if only the trouble was taken to look for it.

A user-centred approach to mental health care provision necessitates the collation of such views along with their complexity since within that complexity lies the answers to why users believe certain issues are more important than others and why they happen to be annoyed about, for example, the behaviour of the psychiatrist they saw. We need to know how users evaluate and that requires an investigation of the totality of the experience of becoming ill, deciding to see a GP and subsequently seeing a mental health professional. Such an investigation demands, at least initially, qualitative research. To this degree the historical accounts we began with perhaps provide more insights than many of the satisfaction surveys currently being used.

Methodology

Location of study

The research problem formulated was how service users evaluate the care that they receive. To answer this question a research project was set up in 1992 with the cooperation of mental health professionals in the Aberconwy and North Clwyd Community Mental Health Teams (CMHTs) in North Wales.

Almost all research in this area to date has been satisfied with identifying users' views of service provision without identifying how those views were arrived at. As such, quantitative research techniques have been deemed theoretically appropriate since the data required were essentially descriptive in nature. Since the research question of how evaluations take place is one of exploration a qualitative approach was deemed most appropriate.

Pilot interviews

To clarify the research problem and highlight some of the issues involved, a small pilot study was undertaken which consisted of in depth unstructured interviews with seven users with at least one episode of inpatient care and a history of contact with mental health services of over three years. Further interviews with three users currently seeing members of the CMHTs, but with no prior contact with mental health services, also took place.

Interviews lasted for approximately one to one and a half hours and covered users' general and specific views regarding their experiences of mental health care. Issues surrounding the research problem were clarified and a clear distinction noted between the types of comments made by new referrals and those made by long term users with inpatient experience.

The main research project

From the pilot interviews the role of past experience in users' evaluations appeared crucial (see below). On this basis it was decided to concentrate the main body of the research on those new referrals to the CMHTs with no prior contact with mental health professionals and no inpatient experience. A further criterion for selection excluded those new referrals who, from the information provided to the CMHTs in the GP's referral letter, appeared to have a psychotic disorder; in reality this excluded very few.

Users were interviewed once prior to their first appointment with a psychiatrist and once one to two weeks afterwards. Those users with subsequent appointments with a psychiatrist were interviewed again between three and four months later. This approach allowed an

240

investigation of the way in which views and evaluations take place and develop; in particular, the role of prior expectations and beliefs were explored. At the time of writing twenty four indepth interviews with fourteen new referrals have taken place. Interviews were attempted with all new referrals meeting the above criteria. However, consent from the service user and the GP had to be gained and an interview arranged prior to the first appointment with the psychiatrist. This severe time restriction resulted in interviews taking place with one third of those eligible.

For these interviews the following topics were covered:

1) Lay health beliefs regarding the nature, cause and cure of their 'illness'.

2) Why the decision to seek help was taken.

3) Views on the treatment provided by the GP and the decision to refer on to the CMHT.

4) Hopes and concerns regarding seeing a mental health professional.

5) Subsequent views on the care provided by CMHTs.

All interviews were tape recorded and transcribed. From this data source users' views of service provision were analysed. The analysis for this chapter draws on data from both the pilot interviews and those from the main body of the research. In total this amounts to thirty four indepth interviews with seventeen new referrals and seven users with inpatient experience. At the time of writing the research is ongoing with a targeted sample size of forty new referrals.

The analysis aimed to generate grounded theory based on a constant comparative method as outlined by Glaser and Strauss (Glaser and Strauss, 1968). Transcripts were examined and coded inductively for categories of concerns distinguished by users as opposed to the researcher (ie. they were developed a posteriori). As each interview was analysed the categories were modified to a slightly higher level of abstraction. However, it should be stressed that this proved minimal since the similarity between users' concerns was strong. The categories of concern outlined below are essentially descriptive and have good descriptive and conceptual validity.

Users' views and level of experience

The nature and content of users' views varies with the level of past experience, particularly whether the user has received treatment as an inpatient. Two main differences are apparent between newcomers to community mental health services and those with past hospital experience. Firstly, while both groups have criticisms of the care that they receive

241

those from newcomers are considerably more difficult to access. Once accessed, however, the reason for this difficulty becomes apparent.

When unsatisfactory events occur new referrals tend to attribute them to factors outside of the health professionals' control and are therefore seen as 'inevitable'. Since there is little point in criticising something which is inevitable comments are seldom made. Consequently, those comments which are made may take the form of a qualified criticism (ie. a criticism which does not imply blame). With this in mind it could be said that new referrals tend to be more 'forgiving' than long term users. The following is a good example. Here, problems in communication between the psychiatrist and user is attributed to the brevity of a meeting rather than the inability of the psychiatrist.

BW: How clearly did he understand your problem and how you felt about it? You said somewhat unclearly.

PT: Well, I think he understood to the extent that he could in that short period of time so it's not a reflection on him it's the time span.'

A second difference between short and long term users of mental health services concerns the targets of criticism. Newcomers tend to comment on specific issues or events while long term users are more general and may express their views in terms of underlying structural problems or mental health professionals' attitudes.

For new referrals all experiences, whether good or bad, are new and as such there is no way of knowing whether or not they are typical. Since users are generally reluctant to criticise, they are likely to presume the experience was atypical and not indicative of some underlying problem. Consequently, new referrals are more likely to comment only on the specific event. Long term users, or those with hospital experience, are more likely to interpret the event in terms of underlying problems with which they have become aware over time; while the event may be mentioned it will be as an illustration of the problem rather than as the problem itself.

Since the way in which long and short term users evaluate is somewhat different I have dealt with them separately below. However, one issue which is of common interest is the fact that service users, irrespective of experience, tend not to express many of their criticisms to staff or in satisfaction surveys.

An unwillingness to criticise

Consumerism or democratisation in health services is dependent upon service users evaluating the care they receive and being willing to express those evaluations. However, the traditional idea of the passive patient being the good patient operates antagonistically to such a notion.

Most service users tend to allow care to be of very poor quality before expressing dissatisfaction; as one woman commented, 'If it comes to the point that you actually say something it'll be said in a bitter way.' Consequently, in surveys overall satisfaction tends to be high, often over 90%. A review by Lebow (1983) listed the results of over fifty surveys; the average percentage of 'satisfied' patients was 77.5%.

Three reasons for this became apparent in the interviews:

a) *Political* The NHS is often perceived in a different manner to other services. Staff may be seen as operating within constraints outside of their control; this engenders an attitude of 'Well, they would do better if they could.' Consequently, care perceived as poor quality may often be excused on the grounds that it is not the fault of health professionals but rather the responsibility of government.

> Yes, people are less critical, people don't criticize the Health Service. Not that people are less critical but the service is so good - people are understanding about health care because of the situation at the moment - it doesn't get enough support from the government.

Furthermore, the traditional perception of staff is not that of commercially motivated individuals but altruistic and caring professionals. Such an image may itself inhibit complaints or at least result in staff being given the benefit of the doubt when behaviour is ambiguous.

> People aren't critical. The NHS is on the news a lot and most people feel benevolent to the staff. Nurses are seen as angels, that's the image. It's the nature of the service really.

Consequently, when asked whether they would be more critical of private health care which they had paid for directly, the usual answer was 'yes'.

> If I was paying I would feel in more of a position to criticize. For example, the drinks machine was empty and I asked for it to be refilled. They said I would have to wait and I thought that was fine. If it was in a hotel and I went to the reception they'd do it straight away and I'd expect it.

b) *Technical competence.* Medical treatment is perceived as technical and esoteric; when this comes to issues of the mind it often borders on the mystical. A number of users commented on their inability to evaluate such care. However, it was also mentioned that within the psychiatric field the patient was the only person who really knew whether treatment was working. Consequently, users were torn between believing they had no technical expertise and yet being aware that they were the final authority on the efficacy of care.

> Patients don't always understand - but they can evaluate, they know when they are happy. People don't feel they can evaluate - I can but I can't complain.
>
> We don't have the knowledge really; but its commonsense, you can tell if its working. I can tell its right now because I'm feeling so good.

Users with a level of self confidence in relation to mental health care did, however, express some criticisms of technical matters. Consequently, the greatest willingness to complain was amongst those who had an experience of mental health care over a number of years.

c) *Rapport.* Explanations above for an unwillingness to evaluate or express evaluations of care can be applied to non-psychiatric specialties in part. However, one issue appears of greater relevance for psychiatric care. A number of users believed that complaining may interfere with the relationship between themselves and the health professionals involved in their care.

Such an interference is to be avoided since for many users the success of treatment may depend on a good rapport between the parties concerned. Whether complaints do have such an effect is unclear; however, many service users do not perceive the risk of interference as worth taking. Consequently, such a fear may silence the less major complaints.

> I can't complain or say anything... I'm not very good at criticizing - I'd be scared that it would damage my relationship with them.
>
> I was going to write to the newspapers once but was told I'd better not because it might come back on me because of the nurses.

While recruiting service users for these interviews one of the commonest reasons for declining to take part was that they did not want anything they said to get back to the psychiatrist or other professional they were seeing; this was mentioned despite guaranteed anonymity.

d) *Halo effect* Those with limited experience of mental health care tended to be less critical than those with more experience. This may not solely be because they lack the confidence and disillusionment of veterans but that for many individuals new to mental health care they are just glad to be seeing someone at last. A halo effect may exist.

> I think people are less critical. When you are ill you want to see somebody - you're just glad to get help.

> When I first used the service I was really pleased with the amount of care I got. I thought the doctor would tell me I was a neurotic housewife and tell me to go away.

Certainly for those seeking treatment from the CMHTs many issues of poor service quality are probably masked by the uncriticalness resulting from service users just being glad to see someone at last. Calnan (1988b), has suggested that a principle element in user evaluations is the goal of the health seeker; at the first few consultations with a member of a CMHT this is primarily the desire not to be rejected or told they cannot be helped.

> BW: Were you disappointed at all that he (the doctor first seen) didn't manage to sort it out, that he decided to refer you on?
> PT: No. I was pleased I went because I did feel I had overcome a sort of personal hurdle and by admitting that you need help and you hope you won't get sort of a smack round the chops saying pull yourself together, there's nothing wrong with you, and the response was positive. I was happy with my doctor's response to me.

A. Views of users with hospital experience

In this section on the views of those with inpatient experience it is interesting to note that the issues and concerns raised bear a strong similarity to those which we have seen were prevalent in the eighteenth and nineteenth centuries.

1. General respect. It was mentioned earlier that the lack of respect afforded to the certified in the latter two centuries stemmed from a particular perception of what madness entailed. It is, perhaps, inevitable that service users continue to recognise and sense this lack.

> I made a note of something that happened on the ward recently. A nurse said to a patient when getting undressed 'come on don't be naughty, take your tights off, its not nice to keep them on when you are going to bed.' She was treating her like a child - taking the moral high ground. It's not right.
> He refused to treat me as if I had a brain in my head. If a patient shows interest in their care they should be treated with respect - he didn't treat me like a human being.

It was shown earlier how Perceval was continually struggling to maintain his own self image despite the way in which staff treated him as an imbecile (Scull, 1989, p.183). Similar criticisms were made by users in the interviews. Treatment in such a manner, resulting over time in a change in one's self perception is an important aspect of institutionalisation.

2) Wrong diagnoses. West (1976) has shown that service users have few expectations when coming into contact with a health care specialty for the first time. Given time, however, cumulated experience can lead to a confidence to express disillusionment felt with the treatment provided. Some of those with a number of years of experience of mental health care had received various diagnoses. This is an issue, so objective in nature, that it appears to allow the service user to voice their concern openly. A re-diagnosis is one doctor saying another was wrong, it is not the user making the evaluation; consequently, users appear to feel freer to complain.

> I was originally diagnosed as neurotic by one doctor, then schizophrenic by another but now the new doctor says I'm not schizophrenic. I knew I wasn't.
> When in *** I questioned the original diagnosis and asked for a second opinion but the doctor absolutely refused. When re-diagnosed and put on new medication which worked better I felt more able to criticize.

The occurrence of a misdiagnosis might by suspected by the user at the time, but faith in the technical ability of the professionals involved may stem an expression of that. When a re-diagnosis takes place, however, the confidence in that technical ability is undermined and their own opinion gains validity. It is little wonder, therefore, that those with re-diagnoses become more open in their criticisms.

3) Nothing but ill. The issue of behaviour interpreted in terms of the individual's psychiatric condition arose earlier in some of the historical accounts. It appears little might have changed. Those who raised this issue expressed it with considerable anger and frustration. Concerning how her therapist deemed her views invalid one woman commented:

> One time I got really angry at a consultation and left and was on the verge of committing suicide. Looking back I think I wanted to change the system. I talked to my therapist but he put it down to my sensitivity and childhood et cetera.

And another woman.

> He (the psychiatrist) didn't know anything about me. I mentioned my weight problem and he asked me if I ate any biscuits or was a closet drinker or something. I told him I didn't drink and I'd forgotten what chocolate tastes like, and I've put on 3 stone. I told him I didn't go out any more because of my appearance but he told me that it was only me who was letting it take over my life. The phone rang, he didn't answer it and the baby got upset. Three months beforehand the consultant had agreed to put me on some new tablets but this registrar wouldn't agree to it. The eventual letter from the doctor (concerning this consultation) said I was clearly still depressed, angry, uncooperative and wouldn't listen.

One gentleman summed up the problem quite simply, 'You can't speak your mind to the doctor - they'll put it down to some abnormality.' While it is difficult to gauge how widespread an experience this is, it is at least important on the basis of the strength of feelings associated with it. Such anger or frustration is hardly surprising since nothing could be more disempowering than for one's beliefs and behaviour to be seen as entirely the product of, for example, one's depression. To be regarded in such a way is to be seen as a machine controlled solely by some pathological entity; one is no longer a person.

4) Power/fear. The final category of concerns that arose related to the vulnerability and powerlessness felt by inpatients. The fear expressed tended to point to a sense of being out of control of one's environment and 'having to watch one's step'.

> Doctors have such a huge amount of power. He could lock me up if he wanted to. They don't listen. A friend is on section but doesn't know why even after two months. Because she is on section they don't take any notice of her opinion. You can feel very powerless.

and

> People here feel the nurses have a lot of power and won't listen to you. Someone threw a jug of water yesterday and this big nurse came down and put her in an arm lock.

Such a sense of fear or powerlessness may, at least in part, stem from a number of the other problems already mentioned. To be out of control of one's situation is disconcerting; however, if something goes wrong then some service users are afraid to complain in case it is put down to their illness or interferes with their relationship with the health professionals they are seeing. For some, whether justified or not, there remains the fear that to complain or rock the boat might result in sectioning: 'You had to keep quiet otherwise they might lock you up.'

B) Views of new referrals to CMHTs

Relative newcomers to community mental health services have a range of criticisms regarding the quality of the care they receive. Whereas long term users with hospital experience have had time to identify patterns within their experience and thus identify underlying issues, new referrals usually comment on isolated and relatively independent events in an essentially descriptive manner. Few comments are made below since doing so invariably involves speculation as to why the user has made the comment. At this stage such speculation has no foundation other than a highly questionable ability to empathise with an individual who may be greatly distressed and/or anxious.

1) Waiting time for appointments. The vast majority of users did not wish to criticise the amount of time they had to wait for their first appointment. However, when questioned in more detail it was apparent that they thought they should not have had to wait so long, but, since they had 'coped' with it they did not wish to complain. The following is quite typical.

> PT: I've been able to cope so I can cope a little longer. I would have liked to see him the next day but I couldn't.
> BW: You don't feel annoyed or disappointed with the system or having to wait this time?
> PT: Well, not me in particular. I'm sure other people would. If I was in a crisis now I would have been off the edge of a cliff or something, you know... it's becoming harder and harder to cope. It's becoming every day closer and you think, oh I wish it was a bit sooner.'

The experience of having a mental health problem can involve times of crisis and intense emotional discomfort. If the individual happened to be suffering from a physical affliction causing a similar level of discomfort then a visit to a hospital accident and emergency department could perhaps be arranged. However, the perception from the new referral to mental health services is that the GP cannot help (since he/she made the referral) and there is no where else to go.

> PT: I found it frustrating because I desperately needed somebody to talk to so badly at that point and I just found it as frustrating as hell that, you know, whoever you contacted you always had to wait a certain amount of time and I didn't think I could wait.
> BW: Would you have thought about complaining to anybody?
> PT: No. Well, because I sorted it out, I think. But if I hadn't sorted it out then, you know, I might have, I don't know.

2) Privacy. Few service users are happy for others to know that they are seeing a mental health professional, particularly a psychiatrist. Consequently, a greater importance is attached to privacy and confidentiality when being referred to a mental health team than would be attached to a referral to any other specialty. For some users this issue is, literally, more important than being 'cured'; an appointment might well be skipped if a lack of confidentiality is suspected. An example of the type of scenario a user may have to deal with is outlined below; in this case this was the woman's first visit to a psychiatrist's clinic which was being held in a GP's surgery.

> PT: The receptionist came and told this other woman it was her turn to see the GP. But this other woman said she thought I had been waiting longer. The receptionist just said 'Oh no, she's waiting to see the psychiatrist'. I wasn't embarrassed I was bloody annoyed. I was shocked that she could do such a thing.

The reason for privacy having such a high priority attached is explored later.

3) Manner. For new referrals to the CMHT a first appointment can be a harrowing experience. Individuals may be very nervous and anxious, not knowing what to expect and fearing being told to 'pull themselves together'. Consequently, many users are quite sensitive to the interaction between themselves and the mental health professional they are seeing. Things can of course go wrong. Some comments could, quite easily, be put down to 'over sensitivity' (not that they are any less important because of that); others, however, are more objectively measurable.

> PT: I wasn't offered a cup of coffee or tea. The psychiatrist walked in with a cup of tea in his hand which s/he'd just made and asked the other psychiatrist if s/he would like a cup. I looked at them and they never said a word. It would have been nice to have a hot drink. You know when you're shaking and you feel it's nice to have a hot drink and your mouth is dry. It would have been nice to be offered.

and:

> PT: I found his mannerisms a little bit...um, unprofessional, that's too hard a word to use. I don't know. For example, now you're sitting forward talking to me and that body language tells me you're interested in what I'm saying. He sat like this, with his legs crossed, arms out like he was sitting on a sofa and I thought, make yourself comfortable! I'm sitting here on the edge of my seat so tense. I felt like saying 'why don't you sit up straight as you're supposed to be a consultant psychiatrist.

4) Impersonal. A number of comments were made which appear to be related to being treated as yet another patient on a never ending conveyor belt.

> PT: I didn't have an opportunity to say a lot. She wanted to know my age, where I came from, how many children I've got, if I'm married, exactly what happened to me, and so on. She was writing down as I was speaking. She just looked at me and wrote it like a robot... I could have sat in front of a computer and punched out that information rather than a person.

> PT: At the start he was extremely professional in the other way. I mean what he was saying, but his mannerisms were 'I've done this before; I know what to do; just keep quiet' and at one point he cut me short.

> PT: We were all in blocks, you know. We're all little blocks and you fit into this block and you fit into that block.
> BW: So you felt more that they were trying to categorise you rather than find out fully how you saw the problem?

249

PT: Yes, definitely, both of them. The first psychiatrist I saw and then Dr G. Both of them put me into a little category.

The process of evaluation - a case study

Qualitative research as above has an advantage over quantitative techniques in that users are enabled to comment on those issues or areas of concern which are important to them rather than the researcher or policy maker. The categories above have good descriptive and conceptual validity; however, they are essentially atheoretical and lack what Rose has termed external theoretical validity (Rose, 1982). Such descriptive views are of limited use for policy making decisions since they represent what users think without explaining why they think it.

If community based services are to effectively differentiate themselves from traditional hospital care they must become responsive to user opinion. This must begin by gaining an understanding of the totality of service users' experience: not simply what their views are but why they hold these views, only then can problems be effectively addressed.

The interviews and the subsequent constant comparative analysis, therefore, goes beyond identifying areas of concern salient to the user and explores the reason for these concerns and their origin. New concepts emerged and are being refined as the research continues. These concepts are inevitably of a higher level of abstraction but have greater explanatory power; for this reason they also have better external theoretical validity and are more useful for enabling users' concerns to be effectively addressed.

Since the research is currently ongoing and thus the concepts and theory not fully developed it is hoped that the following case study demonstrates the importance and usefulness of identifying the way in which evaluations take place. Areas of concern are mentioned throughout but are related to prior beliefs and expectations (notably lay health beliefs) suggesting ways in which concerns can be addressed in a manner purely descriptive comments cannot. If mental health professionals understand how service users evaluate, what views they have, why they hold them and how they can influence subsequent behaviour then services can become truly user-centred.

Background

This woman is married and in her late twenties. She lives in a relatively small community, but is not originally from the area. She experienced a number of traumatic events during childhood and has been aware of a problem with premenstrual syndrome (PMS) for some time.

A) Views prior to first consultation

Lay health beliefs

This woman saw her depressed feelings as the outcome of a struggle between stressful events and her own inner resistance. She held the view that she should be able to deal or 'cope' with these feelings herself without having to see an 'outsider'. These two aspects define a 'strong' person:

1) *Resistance* One's ability to experience traumatic or stressful events without subsequent negative feelings.
2) *Resilience* One's ability to bear or cope with negative feelings once they have arisen.

The situation is seen to be aggravated by the existence of PMS.

> PT: Things just happen to me that are not in my control and that's what causes my depression...also, like I said before, PMS comes into it quite strongly. That's why I'm seeing a gynaecologist.
> BW: So you think it's a number of factors then?
> PT: Oh yes. In my case that is. In another it could be a death. I mean that's something they can't help, a death... Some people are stronger than others. I suppose its just that some people cannot handle certain things and something can trigger something off in the mind, such as death.

It was not the existence of depressed feelings that implied to this woman that she was 'weak' or a 'failure' but the fact that she could not 'cope' with them. Failing to cope was defined as 'seeing someone outside the family'.

> PT: It's all my fault. Why is it other people can cope and I can't. That's how I look at it. I just think to myself why is it my brother and sister have been able to cope? I mean we went through all sorts. Why is it I'm the one who has to go and see a psychiatrist? I know they haven't had things done to them that I have but why do I need to see someone outside the family I just think that if I was a different person I would be able to cope like many, many other people do. They've had things in their past... I've had four major things in my life but I just feel I'm weak. That's the way I look at it.

Consequently, the price of seeking help was, unfortunately, an admission to herself that she could not cope and therefore that she had failed.

Beliefs regarding psychiatrists

Since this woman saw depression as essentially non-biological it is not surprising that the treatment she expected was also non- biological.

251

BW: What would be your ideal meeting with the psychiatrist? What would you say and what would he or she say?

PT: Um, I would say all the things I have been waiting to say. I'd expect him to say something like may be you need hypnotherapy or something, you know - to take you back because there are so many things, because of abuse and things, I've blocked out and I don't remember and I don't want to remember.

There was also some confusion as to the relevance of a biological cure for a non-biological problem; the conclusion was that any drugs would only address the symptoms rather than the cause.

Decision to seek help

This woman's health beliefs regarding depression explain why her request to see a psychiatrist was regarded, by herself, as an admission of her own weakness; it was, therefore, a very difficult decision. The decision to seek help might be characterised as a weighing up of the benefits of seeking help (sorting out the problem) with the costs (admission of failure).

Concerns

When interviewed prior to her first meeting with the consultant psychiatrist a number of salient issues were mentioned which she was worried about; these stemmed from the underlying beliefs outlined above.

1) Privacy

This was a major concern. Since the decision to seek help from a psychiatrist symbolised personal weakness it was important that no-one else knew about it.

BW: So you'd be worried about other people looking at you and thinking you're a weak person and this sort of thing?

PT: Yes, I would. Not so much weak as mentally weak, you know, that I didn't have the ability to cope, that I had to go and see someone. I couldn't talk to may be a friend. Well, it's gone beyond that now. I need to see a psychiatrist so its serious business.

2) Empathy

This consisted of two elements. Firstly there was concern over whether the psychiatrist would realise how bad she really felt and secondly, whether he/she would view her as a failure. On the basis of her health beliefs it is apparent that these two issues are interlinked. She saw that her decision to seek help would be seen as her own inability to cope with either severe or non severe feelings of depression. If the psychiatrist saw her feelings of depression as severe her inability to cope would be justified; if, however, the severity was not recognised then her inability to cope would not be seen as justified, she would be seen as 'weak'.

3) Hope

Since the decision to seek help symbolised weakness it was put off until the depression was very severe and the individual could see no end. Consequently, the fear of being told by the psychiatrist that nothing can be done when one has already admitted that one cannot carry on as things are is quite great.

> PT: But as a psychiatrist I finally think I've got to the top of the pyramid. I've seen all the little people underneath, now I've got to the main man, ha ha.
> BW: So you've got quite a bit at stake here?
> PT: Yes, if he can't sort me out I am lost. I'm going to be this miserable person for the rest of my life.

B) Views after the first consultation

1) Privacy

This woman saw her privacy infringed almost immediately: she was seen by someone other than the named person on the appointment card and had her name called out publicly.

> PT: I saw a woman psychiatrist which threw me because I had been told I was seeing Dr*****. I did mind actually because it meant another person knowing my business - my secrets. I mean I don't think I would have minded so much had I been told beforehand. This woman just came and there was somebody else in the room where I was waiting and she called my name, my full name, which I minded as well. I'm there to be seen by a psychiatrist and she's calling me by my full name. I did tell her at the time... She just said 'why?' I thought, well being a psychiatrist you would have understood.

2) Empathy

This woman had assumed that psychiatrists were not only experts in addressing mental health problems but also 'understood' how people with disorders felt about them, their concerns, hopes and anxieties etc. It appeared that these expectations were so strongly assumed that the user herself was only aware of them when they failed to be met. In addition to having to justify her desire for privacy on two occasions she also made the following comments:

> PT: He was not as sympathetic as I thought he would be after what I had been through... I mean he should realise that I've come through all these things and I've come to see him at this late stage in my life where I think - you know - he must realise that I'm feeling apprehensive... I'm not going to understand everything clearly straight away. He suggested something to me and I said 'Well, how would I do that?', not meaning you haven't told me, and he said 'Well, if you will let me finish'. His hand movement and everything was quite harsh and it just took me back a bit and I thought that's not very nice.

This woman's original fear concerning empathy was that the psychiatrist would fail to realise how bad she felt and/or imply that she was weak. Unfortunately, this concern was fulfilled in what was probably a rather confused interaction.

> PT: They think it's more unhappiness than depression, and they kept saying this actually.
> BW: You look like that confused you.
> PT: Yes, it did because I thought I know what I feel like and, alright, I'm unhappy but I know I'm depressed. I know it. You know, I'm in the situation, I should know what I'm feeling. But they kept saying 'we think you need counselling because you're unhappy because of the things that have happened to you, more than you are depressed.' I'm unhappy but I'm also depressed.
> BW: What would you say the difference was between being unhappy and being depressed?
> PT: Um, I can be unhappy, you know, if it rains when I want to out. I'm unhappy that it's raining. You don't get depressed because it's raining - it's a completely different mood. It's much worse. It's a black, black mood where you can't see an end... They misunderstood me, definitely.

3) Hope

While the psychiatrist was viewed as doing as much as he could this user was disappointed. She had expected some form of treatment which delved into her mind to remove the root problem. This was not offered. However, these comments were made in the form of a qualified criticism; since the psychiatrist was technically competent and did his best he could not be criticised.

> BW: Are you more confident than you were before?
> PT: I'm less confident now I've seen him. I was expecting a lot more when I went to see him. I was expecting...I don't know, I don't know what I was expecting but I was expecting a lot more than I got. I am

254

confident that things will - they will help me as much as they possibly can and I feel they're going to do this counselling business again but I've been through all that... If he doesn't come up with the goods I don't know where I'm going to go.

Summary

It is apparent that this service user had a range of concerns prior to the first consultation, the majority originating in her own health beliefs. Had these beliefs been known to the psychiatrists involved some of the criticisms made could have been avoided. Besides these apparent concerns were a set of expectations so strongly assumed to be correct that they were latent in nature and only revealed when transgressed. In particular it was assumed that psychiatrists would recognise and appreciate a service user's desire for privacy and that she would be treated and respected as an individual as opposed to 'just another person with depression'.

Conculsion

Those with past inpatient experience have different views on service provision from those who have been newly referred to community mental health services. The criticisms of the former include a general lack of respect, frequent re-diagnoses, the removal of their ability to complain by viewing complaints as 'symptoms', and finally a sense of powerlessness resulting in fear. These views are strongly held and are based on a wealth of past experience; consequently, any reorientation of service provision may take a considerable amount of time to improve the views of such users. These concerns must be fully researched and addressed if the moving from hospitals to new community mental health services is to truthfully represent a new regard for the service user. The history of hospital provision and the lessons we can learn from it lie in the memories and experiences of those who were treated there.

New referrals to community mental health services have a host of beliefs about psychiatrists and the nature of mental disorders which manifest themselves implicitly in users' concerns, hopes and anxieties about seeing a mental health professional. These beliefs and concerns interact with the reality of service provision (behaviour of health professionals and the organisation of the service) to produce disillusionment or satisfaction. The outcome may include criticisms regarding waiting times, privacy, health professionals' manner and the impersonal nature of the service.

Most community services are now engaged in collating user opinion about the services provided. However, when ad hoc quantitative techniques are employed users are often asked to reply in simplistic terms to questions about those aspects of care assumed by providers to be important. While qualitative research can solve this problem by enabling users to set the agenda the data invariably remain at a descriptive level. The examples cited earlier indicate that descriptive data can be useful; however, if we have no idea how those views are arrived at it is difficult to know what form solutions should take or where they should be directed. Furthermore, a knowledge of how users evaluate, the nature of their lay health beliefs, and their concerns and anxieties is useful in helping mental health professionals empathise with service users, thus preventing problems before they arise.

The earlier case study demonstrates that it is possible to identify the cause of users' concerns. The intention of the research was to explore and generate theory to explain users' views in a form which facilitates the reorientation of service provision. While the case study has pointed towards the benefits to be reaped, the research as a whole has yet to be completed. However, it is apparent that the role of lay health beliefs and past experiences of mental health care are both crucial to the evaluative process.

Further research in this area is crucial if the resources currently being poured into surveys of user opinion are to have a significant and beneficial effect on services. By using quantitative techniques to access opinion at a descriptive level there is a strong possibility that the contractual obligation to collate user opinion is being fulfilled without any significant changes to service provision.

Community care - The solution?

So many complaints have been made about the institutionalisation engendered by the big psychiatric hospitals that it appears community care cannot fail to improve on the status quo. However, it is unclear how great an improvement community care will produce. The move away from the big asylums is a move away from institutionalisation. Consequently, we might expect community care to reassure users of the validity of their opinions and not to treat them like children or view their complaints as the product of their disorder. To regard an individual's voice as less valid because he or she is receiving mental health care is surely a major factor in the institutionalisation process. To be convinced that one's own opinion is invalid is to be dependent on others.

The genre of institutionalisation mentioned in the interviews appears to be subtle and related to people's attitude to the 'mentally ill' rather than to any geographic basis of care. Consequently, such a process can occur within community based services. While one of the stated aims of community care is to give 'people receiving help a greater say in what is done to help them..' (HMSO, 1988) it will be extremely difficult to ensure that policy changes inform the everyday and mundane ways in which health professionals interact with those with psychiatric disorders.

The crucial question facing new community services is whether in twenty or thirty years time they will have produced service users with criticisms similar to those long term users have now. If the reorientation of services proves successful it will be dealing with critical consumers as opposed to disillusioned patients.

Community services which are committed to improving the views of service users face the challenge of identifying and addressing a host of latent issues. The first stage in such a process is to give users a voice and not just a questionnaire. Service users wish to be listened to and have their views regarded with the same validity as anyone else. This might prove a controversial and problematic area; however, it can be the only starting point for a truly consumer-oriented service.

References

Calnan, M. (1988a), 'Lay Evaluation of Medicine and Medical Practice: Report of a Pilot Study', *International Journal of Health Services* 18:311-322.

Calnan, M. (1988b), 'Towards a Conceptual Framework of Lay Evaluations of Care', *Social Science & Medicine* 9:927-933.

De la Rive, G. (1798), 'Lettre adressee aux redacteurs de la Bibliotheque britannique sur un nouvel etablissement pour la guerison des alienes', in Jones, K. (1955), *Lunacy, Law and Conscience: The Social History of the Care of the Insane*. London: Routledge and Kegan Paul.

Fitzpatrick, R. and Hopkins, A. (1983), 'Problems in the Conceptual Framework of Patient Satisfaction Research: An Empirical Exploration', *Sociology of Health & Illness* 5:297-311.

Gabe, J. and Lipshitz-Phillips, S. (1984), 'Tranquilisers as Social Control', *Sociological Review* 32:524-560.

Glaser, B. G. and Strauss, A.L. (1968), *The Discovery of Grounded Theory*. Chicago: Aldine.

Hayes Newington, H.F. (1886), 'Journal of Mental Science 32', HMSO (1984), *NHS Management Enquiry*. London: HMSO.

HMSO (1988), *Community Care: Agenda for Action*. London: HMSO.

HMSO (1989), *Working for Patients*. London: HMSO.

Lebow, J. L. (1983), 'Research Assessing Consumer Satisfaction With Mental Health Treatment: A Review of Findings', *Evaluation and Program Planning* 6:211-236.

Locker, D. and Dunt, D. (1978), 'Theoretical and Methodological Issues in Sociological Studies of Consumer Satisfaction with Medical Care', *Social Science and Medicine* 12:283-292.

MacKenzie, C. (1985), 'Social Factors in the Admission, Discharge, and Continuing Stay of Patients at Ticehurst Asylum', 1845-1917, in Bynum, W.F., Porter, R., and Shepherd, M. (eds.),*The Anatomy of Madness: Essays in the History of Psychiatry*. London: Tavistock.

Porter, R (1987), *A Social History of Madness*. London: Weadonfeld and Nicolson.

Rose, G. (1982), *Deciphering Sociological Research*. London: Macmillan.

Scull, A. (1989), *Social Order/Mental Disorder : Anglo-American Psychiatry in Historical Perspective*. London: Routledge.

Shyrock, R.H. (1979), *The Development of Modern Medicine*. Madison: University of Wisconsin Press.

Smith, S. (1814), 'An Account of the York Retreat', *Edinburgh Review* 23:189-98.

West, P. (1976), 'The Physician and Management of Childhood Epilepsy', in Wadsworth, M. and Robinson, D. (eds.) *Studies in Everyday Medical Life*. London: Martin Robertson.

Williams, B. (1994), 'Patient Satisfaction: A Valid Concept?' *Social Science and Medicine* 38, 4:509-516.

Index